A Survivor's Guide to Triple Negative Breast Cancer

All You Need to Know from Diagnosis to Treatment, Recovery, and Beyond.

Michele Solak-Edwards

Surviving Triple Negative Since 2016

Copyright © Michele Solak-Edwards 2022

The right of Michele Solak-Edwards to be identified
as the author of this work has been asserted by her in
accordance with the Copyright, Design and Patents Act 1988

All rights reserved. No parts of this publication
may be reproduced or transmitted in any form or by any means,
electronic or mechanical, including photocopy, recording or
any information storage and retrieval system, without
permission in writing from the author.

Hardback (Special Edition with Pink Ribbon) ISBN 978-1-7396328-0-9
Hardback ISBN 978-1-7396328-4-7
Paperback Colour ISBN 978-1-7396328-1-6
Paperback Black & White ISBN 978-1-7396328-2-3
Ebook ISBN 979-1-7396328-3-0

A catalogue record for this book is available from
the British Library

Every effort has been made to contact copyright holders.
However, the author will be glad to rectify,
in future editions, any inadvertent omissions
brought to their attention.

The information in this book has been compiled by way of general guidance, in relation to the specific subjects addressed. This book is not intended to be a substitute, or to be relied on, for medical, healthcare, pharmaceutical or other professional advice, on specific circumstances and in specific locations. Please consult your GP and/or medical team(s) before changing, stopping, or starting any type of medical treatment or alternative therapy. So far as the author is aware, the information contained in this book is correct as at January 2022. Practices, treatment regimes, laws and regulations change, and the reader should obtain up to date professional advice on any such issues. The author disclaims, as far as the law allows, any liability arising directly or indirectly from the use, or misuse, of the information contained in this book.

Dedication

This book is dedicated to my husband Can, daughter Katya, brother Justin, and best friend Nicki, who carried me through my cancer diagnosis and picked me up when I fell.

To my parents, watching from above, from whom I've inherited resilience and strength, I shall be forever grateful.

To my surgeon, James Harvey, who gave me hope when I thought there was none.

And lastly, to all the amazing women I've met on my Triple Negative voyage – keep strong and never give up.

Acknowledgements

I would like to thank three experts in the field of breast cancer for their time and patience in reviewing the medical data in this book, fitting it around their busy professional careers:

- Mr James Harvey, MBBS, FRCS Ed. PhD – Consultant Oncoplastic Breast Surgeon and Reconstruction Specialist
- Professor D. Gareth Evans MB BS MD FRCP FLSW FRCOG ad eundem – Professor and Consultant in Medical Genetics and Cancer Epidemiology
- Professor Andrew M Wardley MBChB MRCP MSc MD FRCP – Global Breast Cancer Oncologist, Medical Director of NIHR / CRUK, Christie Research Facility, Government Advisor, Co-Founder and CEO at Outreach Research & Innovation Group

I would also like to thank Emma Wright, Shannon Healy, Angela McConnachie and Annabel Chown for sense checking and proofreading endlessly, and all the ladies who kindly contributed their time, by putting together their personal stories of reconstruction and surviving after Triple Negative.

The team at Dash Media for bringing my dream of writing a book to life, and lastly, to everyone who has encouraged or taught me something - I heard it all (well, most of it), and this book is for you.

Contents

Preface 1

CHAPTER 1 5
  MY STORY 5

CHAPTER 2 23
  HOW IS BREAST CANCER DIAGNOSED? 23
    What Are The Signs Of Breast Cancer? 25
    What Happens At A Breast Clinic? 26
    I Have Triple Negative Breast Cancer – What Now? 29

CHAPTER 3 32
  UNDERSTANDING BREAST CANCER 32
    What is Breast Cancer? - The Scientific Bit 32
    What Causes Breast Cancer? 35

CHAPTER 4 39
  UNDERSTANDING THE BASICS OF YOUR BREAST CANCER 39
    Where is Breast Cancer or Changes found in your Breast? ... 40
    Explaining Invasive Breast Cancer 41
    Invasive Ductal Cancer (IDC) 42
    Invasive Lobular Carcinoma (ILC) 42
    Pre-cancerous Cells 43
    Ductal Carcinoma in Situ (DCIS) 43
    Lobular Carcinoma In Situ (LCIS) 44
    Analysing DCIS/LCIS 45
    How does Breast Cancer spread to other areas? 46
    Sentinel and Axillary Nodes 46
    Lymphovascular Invasion (LVI) 48

CHAPTER 5 49
STAGES OF BREAST CANCER 49
Stage 0 51
Stage 1 51
Stage 2 51
Stage 3 52
Stage 4 54
TNM staging 55

CHAPTER 6 57
GRADES OF BREAST CANCER 57
What does Grading mean? 57

CHAPTER 7 59
TYPES OF BREAST CANCER 59
Hormonal Breast Cancers (ER+, PR+ and HER2+) 60
Triple Negative Breast Cancer 61
Types in a Bit More Scientific Detail 63
How do I know what type of Breast Cancer I have? 65
Getting Technical – Special Types of Breast Cancer 67
Very Technical – Sub Types of Triple Negative 72

CHAPTER 8 77
EMOTIONS 77
Feelings at Diagnosis 77
Friends and Family 82
Body Image 91
When Things Go Wrong or Not to Plan 93
Delays in Treatments 93
Scans 93
Not being heard or listened to 94

CHAPTER 9 96

PREPARING FOR CHEMOTHERAPY & SURGERY 96

Things to Do Quickly 96

- Eyebrows 96
- Teeth 98
- Thermometer 98
- Visit Your GP 98
- Free Chemotherapy Kit 99
- Pillows For After Surgery 99
- Bedding/Pillow Covers 100
- Bras to Wear After Surgery 100
- Hair 101
- Supplements 102
- Headwear – Turbans, Scarves, Wigs, Hats etc. 102
- Nails 102

CHAPTER 10 103

QUESTIONS TO ASK YOUR ONCOLOGIST/SURGEON 103

Your First Meeting 103

- Questions for your Oncologist: 103
- Questions for your Surgeon: 106
- When am I classed as cancer free? 107
- Copy Letters / Reports 109

CHAPTER 11 110

SURGERY OR CHEMOTHERAPY FIRST? 110

- Surgery before Chemotherapy (Adjuvant) 110
- Chemotherapy before Surgery (Neo-Adjuvant) 111

CHAPTER 12 112

SHOULD YOU HAVE CHEMOTHERAPY? 112

Chemotherapy Isn't Just for the Tumour 113
What If I Only Have A 3-8% Benefit If I Have Chemotherapy?...114
Will Chemotherapy Prevent Recurrence/ Recurrence Statistics?.118

CHAPTER 13 121

CHEMOTHERAPY 121

Typical Chemotherapy Regimes 123
FEC/EC/AC (Anthracycline) Chemotherapy 124
Docetaxel, Paclitaxel, Abraxane & Carboplatin Chemotherapies 126
Typical timescales for chemotherapy 128
What if Chemotherapy Doesn't Work/Only Partly Works? 129
Capecitabine (Xeloda) 131
Before Your First Chemotherapy Session: 133
How is Chemotherapy Given to a Patient? 133
Differences Between PICC and Portacaths 134
Portacath (Power Port / Port) 135
PICC Line 137
Removing the Lines 139
Steroids 139
Common Chemotherapy Side Effects 140
G-CSF Injections – Neutropenia 141
Damage to Veins 142
Nausea 143
Peripheral Neuropathy 144
Other common side effects 145
Chemotherapy is your friend, not your enemy! 150
What to Wear On the Day of Chemotherapy 152
Travelling To Your Chemotherapy Session 153
What to Take On the Day of Chemotherapy 153

What to Eat/Avoid During Chemotherapy 154

Sex and Cancer Treatments 155

Exciting Treatment Advances: 156

Pembrolizumab (Keytruda) Immunotherapy 156

CHAPTER 14 159

IMMUNOTHERAPY 159

CHAPTER 15 162

SURGERY 162

Different Main Types of Surgery: 163

Lumpectomy – Wide Local Excision 165

What Will My Scars Be Like? 167

Will a Lumpectomy Change How My Breast Looks? 167

What Are the Advantages of a Lumpectomy? 168

What Is Surgery Like for a Lumpectomy? 168

Mastectomy 171

No Reconstruction after Surgery 174

General Surgery Information 175

What to Take on the Day of Surgery 175

Surgery Complications 177

Seroma 177

Lymphoedema 178

Necrosis 180

Aching, Numbness, Tingling and Shooting Pains 180

Pulmonary Embolism (PE) 181

New Lumps or Bumps 182

Ongoing Pain in the Breast Area 183

Cording after Node Removal 183

CHAPTER 16 185

DIFFERENT TYPES OF BREAST RECONSTRUCTION 185

Implant Reconstruction 185

DIEP Reconstruction 188

Latissimus Dorsi Reconstruction (LD) 190

Transverse Upper Gacilis Reconstruction (TUG) 191

Other Types of Reconstruction 192

Nipple Reconstruction 192

CHAPTER 17 195

PATIENTS' STORIES OF SURGERY 195

Lumpectomy Surgeries 195

Michele's Story – Lumpectomy with Sentinel Node Removal 195

Cheryl's Story – Lumpectomy with Full Node Removal 200

Natalie's Story – Lumpectomy/Node Removal Using One Scar .. 203

Kalie's Story – Lumpectomy - Invasive Lobular & DCIS 205

Melanie's Story – Lumpectomy to Mastectomy - ER+ to Triple Negative 208

Mastectomy Surgeries with Reconstruction 213

Michele's Story – Double Mastectomy - Immediate Implants 213

Vicki's Story – Double Mastectomy - Immediate DIEP 219

Di's Story – Double Mastectomy - Immediate DIEP 226

Carley's Story – Double Mastectomy - Immediate TUG 232

Kath's Story – Double Mastectomy - Immediate LD 237

Mastectomy Surgeries with No Reconstruction 240

Sheila's Story – Single Mastectomy with No Reconstruction 240

Lisa's Story – Single Mastectomy with No Reconstruction 242

Jo's Story – Single Mastectomy with No Reconstruction 245

CHAPTER 18 247

RADIOTHERAPY 247

Side Effects 250

Changes to Skin Appearance 250
Tiredness and Weakness 251
Swelling of the Breast 251
Loss of Hair to Armpit 252
Restricted Movements to Arm and Shoulder 252
Long Term Side Effects and Complications 252

CHAPTER 19 254

HAIR 254

All about Hair 254
When Will I Lose My Hair? 254
Cold Capping 255
Nasal Hair! 261
Eyelashes 261
False Eyelashes 262
Eyebrows 264
Alternative Head Wear 265
Wigs 266
How to Buy a Wig: 267
Wig Caps 269
What to Look For in a Wig 270
Taking Care of Your Wig: 272
Wig Stands 274

What About After Treatment Ends? 274

Hair Extensions / Systems 274
Colouring Your Hair 275

CHAPTER 20 277
BISPHOSPHONATES... 277

CHAPTER 21 281
TEETH 281
Why Can Treatment Affect My Teeth?.............................282
What Can I Do to Avoid Dental Problems? 282
Accessing Dental Care and Dental Costs 283

CHAPTER 22 286
GENETIC TESTING... 286
The Basics of Genetics and Breast Cancer 286
Genetics in More Detail...289
What if My Health Authority Won't Test Me? 294

CHAPTER 23 296
FERTILITY, PERIODS, MENOPAUSE, HRT, HORMONES . 296
Preserving Fertility 296
Periods 297
Menopause / HRT / Hormones 298

CHAPTER 24 303
YOUR LEGAL RIGHTS / FINANCIAL HELP 303
Employment Rights..303
Returning to Work After Treatment 305
Financial Help...308
Employment Support Allowance.....................................309
Personal Independence Payment (PIP) 309
Housing and Council Tax 311
Travelling Costs 311
Grants 311
Critical Illness Policies 312

Travel Insurance 312
Medical Exemption Form 314
National Toilet Schemes 314

CHAPTER 25 316
AFTER TREATMENT ENDS 316
Aches, Pains, Tiredness and Cognitive Issues 319
Cancer Related Cognitive Dysfunction (Chemo Brain) 321
Anti-Depressant Tablets 323
Counselling 324

CHAPTER 26 327
FUTURE DEVELOPMENTS - TRIPLE NEGATIVE BREAST CANCER 327
Drug Trials 327
Identifying Cancer Cells Before They Show on Scans (ctDNA) ... 329
Zest Trial – ctDNA Monitoring/Parp Inhibitor Treatment 330
PARP Inhibitors 331
Immunotherapy: 332
Trodelvy (Sacitzumab Govitecan) – Antibody Drug Conjugates 332

CHAPTER 27 335
NATURAL / ALTERNATIVE OR COMPLEMENTARY REGIMES 335
LifeMel Honey to Help with Low Neutrophils 335
Diet 337
Alternative/Complementary Regimes 339
Repurposed Drugs 340

CHAPTER 28 342
THINGS I WISH I'D KNOWN AT DIAGNOSIS 342

CHAPTER 29 344
SURVIVOR STORIES... 344
Annabel's Story – Diagnosed 2002..344

Julie's Story – Diagnosed 2009...347

Marian's Story – Diagnosed 2010...348

Lisa's Story – Diagnosed 2003 351

Alison's Story – Diagnosed in 2011..357

Angela's Story – Diagnosed 2010...361

CHAPTER 30 367
WEBSITES AND USEFUL INFORMATION 367
CHAPTER 31 371
GLOSSARY / ABBREVIATIONS... 371
ABOUT THE AUTHOR 380

Preface

They say everybody has a book inside them - I just didn't think the catalyst for mine would be a diagnosis of Triple Negative Breast Cancer! I always imagined writing a book for children or perhaps a science fiction thriller, but never could I imagine typing the words that I'm about to.

So, what's the impetus behind this book? When I was diagnosed, I guess I was like most people, totally clueless that breast cancer isn't just "breast cancer". Who knew there were different types? I hit the internet trying to find answers. BIG mistake. The internet is an amazing place for all else, but when you are diagnosed with cancer, it's probably the last place to go to – But the truth is, I wanted to know what was happening and when? What could I expect? What did I have to do to survive? And more importantly - Was I going to die? I found websites but they tended to cover breast cancer in general, not specifically Triple Negative breast cancer. Moreover, they did not help me to understand the process from start to finish either. I realised that I was clicking through websites and only getting more confused than when I first started searching.

There were some fantastic breast cancer websites but for me, they didn't have the personal touch to guide me from start to finish from a patient's perspective. I found out that with Triple Negative Breast Cancer in particular, the reading can be doom and gloom. On some websites, there were just a few clinical paragraphs, and if you managed to find medical papers, they were crammed full of words I had never seen before and most made really scary reading. It was definitely something you didn't want to read when first diagnosed!

Therefore, the aim of this book is to offer a one-stop-shop to (hopefully) answer questions for anybody diagnosed with Triple Negative Breast Cancer specifically. As a disclaimer I must add that I am not a medical professional. All of the contents in this book are from my own experience. It is quite possible that over time, treatments, and surgeries will change so things might be different in the future from what you read in this book, but for now, it's a good indication of what you may experience. For any scientific data I have provided, I have tried to include images to illustrate and wherever possible, I have broken it down into simpler explanations in the hope of removing a lot of the jargon and making the information on the subject reader friendly. The information provided I hope will give you a head-start if you want to read scientific papers or ask your oncologist for more detail. If you want to research further, I strongly suggest you only refer to reputable websites such as Cancer Research UK, Macmillan, Breast Cancer Now, Prevent Breast Cancer, Team Verrico etc – links to these websites can be found in Chapter 30.

It's important to note that I have written this book specifically for ladies with what's called "primary" early breast cancer. That means cancer may be in the breast and/or nodes in the armpit and hasn't spread to other organs in the body such as the liver, lungs, brain, bones etc (which is known as either a Stage 4 or metastatic breast cancer).

Metastatic cancer is a separate topic, and treatment options differ, so to avoid confusion, this book concentrates on the treatment of early/primary breast cancer. That being said, for somebody newly diagnosed with Stage 4 Metastatic Triple Negative cancer who has never had a primary cancer, the information in this book may well give some useful insights.

I was treated in England and if you live in Scotland, Wales, and Northern Ireland you might find a few differences in timelines and one or two other issues. However, the majority of the four nations do follow a similar route with Triple Negative Breast Cancer so this book will largely cover all the UK.

The first chapter is all about me – very self-indulgent! – But I wanted to detail the emotional roller coaster I went through. Although we all deal with a cancer diagnosis differently, I've had ladies say, "I could have written that myself", so I hope some aspects will resonate with you. Feel free to whizz past that chapter and get to the nitty gritty stuff! I won't be offended!

Having a cancer diagnosis is almost impossible to describe to somebody who hasn't walked in our shoes. Yet I've tried to be honest about how it affected me and how "normal" it can be to totally fall apart, feel helpless and out of control. The chapters in the book detail the various steps I went through, and I've written the book in the order that most people go through treatment. However, even then, the order might vary from case to case. While the information is the same, it is possible you may want to dip into one chapter before another and the book is designed to allow you to do so.

Above all else, I want you to know that there **IS** hope. That you **CAN** beat this and there **IS** life after Triple Negative and, believe it or not, there are quite a few positives to having Triple Negative Breast Cancer! I was treated in 2016 and so far, crossing my fingers, toes, and eyes, I'm still Triple Negative free. The last chapter in this book contains real life stories from Triple Negative survivors who are ten and even twenty years cancer-free after their diagnosis. I hope that their experiences can convince you that there really can be life after Triple Negative.

CHAPTER 1

MY STORY

Before February 2016 my world was pretty much cancer-free. Well, not quite cancer-free, as my grandparents had died of cancer, as did their sisters and brothers. BUT the truth is that they lived in an age when nobody thought that smoking could be harmful and working with asbestos hadn't been identified as a possible risk. Cancer in my family was all different types; although a distant great aunt may have had breast cancer that's been difficult to confirm.

My father was born in 1916 (he was 47 when I was born!) and he was illegitimate, with my grandmother falling pregnant to a soldier on home leave. Sadly, enough, although my father knew that side of his family, it wasn't the "done" thing to be open about the circumstances of his birth. Therefore, he was brought up believing his mother was actually his sister (having a child out of wedlock in 1916 was really taboo) – all very complicated but not unusual for the time. But the reason for this explanation is that one side of my family history is totally unknown. I know my grandfather's name and his brothers' names, but even though I tried to track them down when I was diagnosed to find out more about their medical history, I didn't have much luck. The question was, did they have breast cancer on that side of the family? I have no idea and no way to find out.

My mother's side of the family was much easier to research and document. It was this side that had a depressing amount of cancer of all different types but not much breast cancer.

So, my exposure to, and knowledge of, breast cancer was almost non-existent. I had read in newspapers about Angelina Jolie's elective double mastectomy due to having the inherited defective breast cancer gene that increases the risk of getting breast cancer. However, my knowledge did not extend much further than this - I remember reading her story and how she had taken the decision to have a double mastectomy thinking, "I'd do that if I had breast cancer", but... thinking about it, and living it is a whole different ball game! I never imagined that I could ever be faced with that decision, so it was nothing more than a passing thought.

In January 2013, three months before my 50th birthday a letter dropped through my letterbox explaining I was now part of the NHS breast screening programme due to my age. I remember thinking that it was a gift that I didn't really want for my 50th!

However, I went along, had my first ever mammogram and filled out a long form about my family history about cancer and thought no more of it. Several weeks later, I received a letter telling me that my mammogram was fine, – and then I received another letter inviting me for a smear test. The gifts that kept on coming! Thankfully the results of the mammogram and smear were both clear and showed no issues.

Fast forward three years later to January 2016 another similar letter arrived, inviting me for a mammogram. I made an appointment and went to the mobile scanning unit on the grounds of my local hospital. As I walked towards the unit, I remember wondering how many lives were changed after having a mammogram. It was nothing more than a passing thought, but for some reason, - perhaps gut instinct, it stayed with me.

I had both boobs squashed (which isn't particularly pleasant, but it was over in a few minutes, and I'd go through it all again, every day, if I had to). I was told that a letter would be sent to me in the next couple of weeks with the results. Interestingly, I also remember the radiographer being very business-like and I just had a feeling that she had seen something. I was probably reading too much into it, but it was an odd feeling. Whether she did or didn't, I'll never know, but I couldn't shake off the feeling.

A week after the mammogram, I received a letter from the NHS thanking me for taking part in the survey (the document I had completed three years earlier at my first mammogram!), stating my risk of getting breast cancer was the same (or maybe slightly lower) than the national average, based on the answers I'd provided. I'd completely forgotten even completing the survey 3 years earlier.

Then a few days later, the letter arrived that changed my life. It said that something had been seen on my mammogram and whilst 80% turned out to be nothing, (and might just be some changes due to hormones, or cysts etc), they wanted to investigate a bit further. The letter explained the appointment, in most cases turned out to be nothing, but I had a gut feeling. I knew it was going to be bad news, and I even knew that the breast affected was my right one. The letter was very positive, and there was nothing to suggest anything sinister, but I couldn't shake off the feeling that I wasn't one of the 80%. I told my husband that I expected bad news, but he shook it off. I knew, and I don't know how. I just knew.

My appointment was scheduled for 2 weeks later at a specialist breast clinic, The Nightingale Centre, in Manchester. My husband had totally forgotten although we had agreed he would come with me. He had already left for work, so I went alone.

The Nightingale is housed in a fairly new building on the grounds of Wythenshawe Hospital and has an impressive reception area but dishearteningly, it's always full of ladies (and I suspect a few men) waiting to be seen.

The letter had outlined the process for that visit which would be another mammogram, possibly an ultrasound and then a meeting with a doctor. So, I wasn't surprised when I was called for my mammogram first. This time the machine was an incredibly and impressively large one, like something out of a sci-fi movie with lights all around. Within 10 minutes I was back in the waiting room for the next step. Waiting outside, I actually felt a deep fear and I was fighting to hold back the tears. I had absolutely no reason to feel like this, and this is coming from someone who had been in and out of hospital for a variety of reasons, always taking things in their stride, but this time just felt different.

I was then called for an ultrasound. I lay on the bed and the radiographer, (that I've since found out is a specialist consultant) told me "something" had shown on both mammograms and that he wasn't particularly concerned but wanted to double-check. All very normal and not alarming.

However, he seemed to take ages scanning, and when he moved the scanner up to my armpit and started looking there, I had a sense that something was wrong. He was taking a very long time looking around. I said to him "You think there's something more to this now, don't you?" and his reply is one I will never forget. He said "I'm 95% certain this is cancer, but I need to take a few biopsies to make sure. Is it okay if I do it now?".

Some people say they hear the words but don't take them in, but that wasn't the case for me. Those words hit me with full force. I felt like I was in another world, and it wasn't happening to me. Perhaps it was a horrible dream and I'd wake up any moment. I started to silently cry because I remember trying to keep it together, but tears were streaming down my face. I agreed to the biopsies, and the radiographer took them – in fact, I think he took two, but it could have been more. He explained it would sound like a click and would be a little painful, but he suggested not to move. He took the biopsies, and it was an odd sensation – a bit like being stapled - and then told me that he had also put in a "marker". It all happened so quickly that I didn't really care what he was doing. I'd just heard "cancer". Cancer. The word nobody wants to hear EVER.

After the biopsies and marker, I was told to get dressed, and the radiographer came back in. He said, "Is there anything you want to ask me?" and I said, "How long have I got – am I going to die?". To my surprise, he smiled and said "No. This is very small, and I think it's been caught early, and your nodes look clear. We've come a long way with breast cancer, and now it's treatable".

I had no idea what nodes meant and I'm not sure I heard that it was small or that it could be treatable. I just heard the word "cancer" going round and round my head. He explained that the biopsies would be sent away, and I'd receive an appointment in a couple of weeks to confirm whether it was cancer or not. Two weeks? TWO WEEKS? Two weeks sounded like a lifetime. What if I DID have cancer? Leaving it in my body for two weeks felt wrong, and very, very, scary. I know now that if it is cancer, typically, you will be having treatment within 4-6 weeks but at the time, the thought of leaving cancer in my body for even one more day was terrifying.

For some ladies, they have a sense of calm, or the diagnosis hits them later, but I think as I was half expecting bad news, it hit me straight away. I was in such a mess that the nurse took me into a side room and gave me a cup of coffee. She also gave me a booklet and explained she would be my breast care nurse. I don't think I heard anything she said either. I felt like I was totally spaced out and that this really wasn't happening. I wanted to wake up or turn back time or anything for this to stop happening.

There I was, on my own, clutching a yellow booklet with tears streaming down my face, and I had to walk out to the car park through the packed reception. Bizarrely, as I walked out of the reception, I wondered if the people in the waiting area knew how my life had just changed. Did they know what the booklet I was holding meant? How many others would walk out of the hospital with a different outcome and feel like they were walking on air with happiness? I tried to keep my head down so people wouldn't notice me.

It sounds dramatic, but my legs were shaking, and I honestly felt I was going to faint as I made my way to the car. Ironically it was a lovely sunny day for March. How could it be sunny when I felt surrounded by a storm? I looked around and people were just carrying on as normal. How could they? It's not a normal day. My world had changed in a way I couldn't understand.

I started to drive home and phoned my husband. I just remember saying "I've got cancer". My husband was shocked and said, "What do you mean you've got cancer?" and I just repeated "I've got breast cancer". I couldn't talk and hung up on him. I got myself home and sat down on the sofa, and two minutes later, my husband came running through the front door. He was in total shock, and also in denial. He kept saying "No you don't have cancer. We've got to wait until the results, but you won't have cancer. It'll be ok" but I knew he was wrong. If a radiographer says they're

95% certain it's cancer, then the likelihood is, it's cancer. A medical professional very rarely says anything like this, so I knew he was right. By the way, I was so glad that he had told me he thought it was cancer, because it gave me time to adjust and, whether this was a blessing or not, do some research.

Then came possibly one of the hardest parts of the processes. Katya is our only daughter, and, at the time, she was 12 years old – a difficult age for any kid. I'd had numerous miscarriages (into double figures) before she arrived so, although she was never spoiled with material things, we spoiled her with love. How on earth were we going to tell her? Should we tell her? Should we wait until we knew more? Katya and I were (and still are), incredibly close, and I knew she'd take one look at me and know something was wrong, so I didn't think not telling her was an option, but I was so conflicted – do we tell her something/anything/nothing? Between us, my husband and I decided to tell Katya the truth but couch it in terms that were positive – along the lines that they'd found something, and there was nothing concrete to suggest at the moment that it was worrying, and I could be treated. We thought being honest with her would be the best way forward. Would I do this again? Yes, I think I would, but it's such a difficult balance, and did have ramifications further down the line, but more of that later.

We arrived at the dance school where Katya was dancing after school, learning a very emotional routine to honour a gentleman who had lost his life in the war. There were lots of parents watching the rehearsals. We sat down but as soon as the music started, I knew I wasn't going to be able to hold it together. I got up and made my way to the toilet, but my legs were shaking, and I was desperately trying to hold back the tears. I'd just got to the toilets when Mags, the receptionist, saw me, and I guess my face said it all because she grabbed me, gave me a hug, and said, "What's wrong?" I dissolved. I couldn't hold it in and said, "I've got breast cancer". Mags just held me. She gave me the longest, best hug ever. She didn't speak, she just held me until I started to compose myself. I had lost my mum when I was pregnant with Katya and even though Mags and I are only separated by a few years in age, her hug was just like having a hug from my mum and it's one I will NEVER forget. I'm typing this with tears running down my face because thinking about it brings back a deluge of emotions. I made her promise not to say anything and got myself together just as my husband (whose name is Can – pronounced Jan) came out with Katya.

When we got home, Katya could sense something was wrong, and I told her we had something to tell her. I've no recollection of what we said or how we said it. I just remember Katya breaking down in floods of tears. Interestingly, she has no memory of that and has denied it happened. I'm pretty sure that from that moment, she protected herself by pretending it wasn't happening. Not in a conscious way, but it was like she just shut everything out so she could carry on as normal. For four years after my diagnosis, if the word "cancer" was mentioned, I literally saw her switch off. It's a bit like if you don't believe something, it's not true. Telling her was one of the hardest things I've ever had to do.

When you're diagnosed with cancer, telling people you love is probably the worst part, because it's not like they can do anything. You're changing their lives for the foreseeable future because you're ill. It made me feel guilty, which is daft because it's not something I had any control over – nevertheless, I felt incredibly guilty.

Between having the tests, and getting a diagnosis was probably the worst time of my life. Don't forget, at this point, the biopsy results weren't in, so all I had to go on were the radiographer's words and my gut feeling, but that was enough. During this time, I felt like I was in a waking nightmare, in limbo with nothing concrete either way. I hit the internet, hard, and everywhere I looked seemed to be negative.

It was also a huge learning curve because I became aware that breast cancer isn't just breast cancer. Who knew!? There are different types – hormone fed breast cancers, some that just affect the skin, and then something called Triple Negative which isn't fed by hormones and from what I read, was associated with a death sentence because it is hard to treat and rare, with only about 15% of breast cancers being Triple Negative. It was awfully confusing. I couldn't really understand what it all meant, terms that I'd never heard before. My head was completely mashed, so rational thought was out of the window. The one thing I knew, was that I didn't want Triple Negative Breast Cancer. I wanted one of the common, more easily treatable ones – one with a "+" after it - but my gut feeling was that when the test results were back, they would tell me it was Triple Negative.

I turned to a friend, Jayne, who had been diagnosed with breast cancer a year before and was just finishing treatment. She spoke at length with me and did her best to reassure me, but all I could think was how ignorant I'd been when she'd been diagnosed. At that time, I had just thought, "Well it's breast cancer, she'll beat this", but now I was walking in her shoes and oh my word, I had had no idea how significant an impact it had made on her when she was diagnosed. I suddenly understood it and felt guilty that I hadn't offered more support to her.

The feeling of impending doom was made worse, not only because of my constant internet searching but because since my appointment at the Nightingale, I hadn't slept. Well, I did sleep, but it was for 10 minutes here and there, and my last thought before going to sleep was "I've got cancer" and the first thought on opening my eyes was "I've got cancer". I dreamed about cancer and dying. My husband told me I cried in my sleep. I cried when I was awake and cried when I was asleep! I was an absolute mess.

What was really odd was that my senses were heightened. I looked at the blue sky, the birds singing, and it was like a weird film where things looked brighter and sharper – I have no idea if that happens to other people and whether it was just from sleep deprivation, but it made me desperately want to stay alive. I didn't want to die. I wanted to see sunrises, sunsets, my daughter grow up, I wanted to laugh again. I definitely didn't want to die, but all I could think about was dying and things I wouldn't see, like my daughter finishing school, going to college, getting married, having children etc

Sure enough, just over a week of sleep deprivation and crying more than I've cried in my entire life, Can and I were sitting in an office at the Nightingale to be told I definitely had breast cancer. Interestingly, I had to ask what type, and to no surprise, it was confirmed that I had Triple Negative!

It was then confirmed that I would need to see a surgeon in the next few weeks to discuss plans. They didn't know if I was having chemotherapy at this point, but I was told that it was highly likely I would. Of course, I asked whether I'd lose my hair – which was the only part of me I really liked – and yes, I probably would. It all seemed so unreal again. So now I knew that I had Triple Negative Breast Cancer and would be losing my hair.

It seemed like I'd received a death sentence, and privately, without telling anybody, I started to plan my funeral. I sent a message to my brother (who lives in Switzerland) asking him to promise to look after my husband and daughter if I died. I'm ashamed of sending that message now and have no idea how my poor brother must have felt getting it, but I was desperate. I HAD CANCER, and not any old cancer, I HAD TRIPLE NEGATIVE BREAST CANCER!

If you've not been close to a cancer patient, your only view of what it might be like is what you see in movies or on television. So, I had visions of being bald, looking desperately thin and lying on the bathroom floor with my head down the toilet being sick. The reality is actually very different to that, but I was terrified about what was going to happen.

The wait to see my surgeon was two long weeks. Two weeks feel like an eternity when you're still not sleeping, internet exhausted, and just want the cancer OUT! So, two weeks later (with still no sleep), I walked like a zombie (with Can, who never left my side at any appointment or chemotherapy appointment after that), into the meeting with my oncoplastic surgeon, James Harvey. I will say without apology, that James Harvey is my hero. He has such a calm way of delivering news – and in a way that you understand what's going on. At our first meeting, he said words that I'll never forget. "You're lucky. This has been caught very early, and it's treatable. If you'd had your mammogram 3 months earlier, the likelihood is, the tumour wouldn't have been seen, and if you'd left it for another 6 months, the outcome might well be different. You're very lucky".

I never thought I'd hear that I was lucky to have cancer, but lucky was a word that stuck with me! I've played the lottery, entered prizes, bought raffle tickets, and never have I been lucky, but hey, I'd been lucky when it counted.

That night I slept like a baby! For the first time, I had a glimmer of hope – maybe I could get through this and, more importantly, survive! Don't get me wrong, there were lots of times after that, when I felt full of utter despair, stopped sleeping again, and had to face my mortality, BUT for the time being, I was much calmer than I had been.

So, what was the plan? At that same meeting, Mr Harvey explained that I needed to have surgery first, and most likely chemotherapy after, so did I want a lumpectomy or mastectomy? Now, this is one of the reasons that I've decided to write this book. A lumpectomy or mastectomy? How on earth could I choose? What did it mean in reality? Do I really have to have one? Why am I even being asked about a mastectomy when I've just been told that my breast cancer has been found early? Will I have no boob on one side? What will the scars look like?

These (and many more questions), passed through my sleep deprived. frightened mind, and I had to make a decision! It's almost impossible, because timelines mean you really need to get cancer out, but you have to make such an important decision quickly. Mr Harvey was fantastic at outlining both procedures, but I still couldn't decide, so I asked him what he would recommend if it was his wife, and he said "lumpectomy". That was fine by me, so lumpectomy is what I chose. I've never regretted that decision, and it was right at the time. Interestingly though, for me, the more I read about Triple Negative, the more I wanted a mastectomy – but not just a single one – a double mastectomy, but more of that later.

To cut a long story short, I had a lumpectomy 2 weeks later, followed by 8 months of chemotherapy and then, 6 weeks later, a double mastectomy. It wasn't easy. Yes, I lost my hair despite using something called a "cold cap" that turned me into a human icicle, but I had to deal with being bald (with a weird, shaped head I never knew I had)! I got seriously ill with Klebsiella Pneumonia halfway through treatment, and I had NO idea how serious it was, until a few months later when my oncologist told me!

I learned so much with every month of my journey and drove my team bonkers by continually asking questions. But that's how I dealt with it. I wanted to know EVERYTHING. I knew knowledge was power, and if I had knowledge, I could then understand what I was dealing with. For some people, they don't want to know – some knowledge can be dangerous – but for me, it was an essential part of dealing with the hand I'd been dealt.

With this knowledge I realised about halfway through treatment that I wanted a double mastectomy. I must stress that this is such an individual decision. For many, this would be something they couldn't even consider. For others an easy decision, but for me, it was a decision that was a slow burner. Bearing in mind I know little about my family history, there is, however, a suggestion of Ashkenazi heritage (genetics that carries a higher risk of breast cancer, usually with the BRCA1 and BRCA 2 genes the same ones Angelina Jolie has), so there was always a question in mind as to whether I may have inherited a risk. I tested negative for BRCA1 and 2 but was never tested further than that.

Also, how I was diagnosed played on in my mind, and I realised just how lucky I had been. I couldn't feel the tumour,

I had no symptoms, and had it not been for the mammogram, I would never have known. The last consideration was that my tumour was one of the fastest growing tumours you can have. So, it was a real issue for me as to how I would know if it happened again, and would I catch it in time? These were risk factors for me, but I need to stress that this is incredibly personal, and I'm not trying to justify or advocate this route for anybody, but I'm aware that if you're reading this book, you may wonder why I converted from a lumpectomy to a double mastectomy.

For all those reasons, I decided to ask my surgeon if he would be prepared to operate again and give me a double mastectomy. I have to say that I was expecting either an outright "No" (as many surgeons will not operate on healthy tissue) or simply a "Yes". But, in truth, I didn't get either! Mr Harvey asked me my reasons, and then gave me some information, and told me to go away, think about it and to see him again if I still wanted it. I think I saw him three times, and each time he asked me more questions, challenging (gently) my thought process, and I'm guessing it was his way of making sure that it was something I really wanted, and not just a whim or knee jerk reaction. After he was convinced, he said I would have to see a psychotherapist and he wouldn't agree to operate until he had seen their report (which was absolutely the correct thing to do). Ultimately, I passed the psychological assessment, and Mr Harvey agreed to the surgery. I have never regretted my decision, and I credit Mr Harvey for ensuring that I had the time and space to think everything through.

If I look back over my whole diagnosis, the worst times for me (emotionally) were before my treatment started, and then after all treatment ended. It's interesting to mention here, that the majority of ladies find after treatment the hardest, because your team has walked away, and your family and friends think you're cured. The reality is that I felt more vulnerable, and alone, than I had ever felt in my life. I was consumed with feelings of dread, and the thought of recurrence or spread to other organs.

Every time I lost a friend from one of the online groups I had joined, I would sink into a terrible low. Having cancer isn't something that you have, and when it's done, you pick up your life where you left off. The reality is that you have a new "normal". Some ladies change their whole lifestyle, others try to keep it the same as before and others even shrink away from life as they find it too difficult to cope.

After 18 months of feeling haunted by the fear of death and cancer returning, I asked my GP to refer me to Macmillan for counselling. It was honestly the best thing I ever did. My counsellor just got me! From our first meeting, she knew what I needed, and I credit her for giving me my sanity back. There is no doubt that I was suffering from Post-Traumatic Stress Disorder (PTSD), and there are occasions when I feel it creeping back, BUT my new normal is now my new normal! I don't say I'm a survivor, because that feels like tempting fate but, if asked, I will say that I am strong, and for now I'm cancer free. Interestingly, when I was nearing the end of writing this book, I tested out titles on fellow Triple Negative ladies, and they all said that they would want to know that I was a survivor, so you'll see that I have used this word and it's even in the title of the book!

It's six years now since I had my Triple Negative tumour, but in 2021 (the horrible year of Covid and Isolation), I was diagnosed with a completely (and totally unrelated), very rare bladder cancer. Trust me to get yet another rare cancer! This one though, is super rare and I'm only number 48 in the world to have this type of cancer. Again, I've been told how lucky I am because I sensed I had cancer, pushed for a scan and there it was. Having cancer, a second time is, of course, a shock, but I am so much better informed now, and have been able to work with my new team in coming up with a plan. Maybe I'll write a book on that one in another 5 years!

For now, though, please, please, please, understand that this is a time in your life that you can never have imagined, but dig deep, stay strong, take all of the treatments thrown at you. Within a year, you'll be coming out the other end. Despite what you think after your diagnosis, you **CAN** do this, and you **WILL**.

CHAPTER 2

HOW IS BREAST CANCER DIAGNOSED?

If you're reading this book, and are interested in Triple Negative Breast Cancer, you've either been diagnosed, know somebody who has, you are in the medical profession, or maybe none of those, but just want to learn a bit more about Triple Negative breast cancer. So, you may, or may not, understand how breast cancer might be found, therefore it's worth expanding here, because early detection is essential.

Typically, there are two main paths that lead to a breast cancer diagnosis, (1) a lump or suspicious sign found by the patient themselves or (2) by a routine check-up or mammogram. Unfortunately, breast cancer can occur at any age, and whilst it's more prevalent in ladies over 40, younger ladies can develop breast cancer too. It's important if you feel that something isn't right, to see your GP. I know that sounds really obvious, but many ladies find a lump, or are worried there's something wrong, but they put off going to see their doctor – usually this is because they don't want to know what it is.

This is something you should never do. Breast cancer, if left to its own devices, won't go away on its own. It will grow, and then potentially spread. How fast can this happen? There's no set time period, and it depends on your individual breast cancer. Some are slow growing, and others have a mission to grow as big as they can, as rapidly as they can.

Any delays in approaching your GP means a delay in diagnosis, treatment, and possibly the outcome, so early diagnosis is key.

Although I would rather not dwell on instances where things go wrong, or don't work out, I think it's important to remember that Sarah Harding (from Girls Aloud), who lost her life to breast cancer, delayed going to see her GP. She admitted she made various excuses, but probably she just didn't really want to know. This is very common. For some ladies (and potentially this includes Sarah), breast cancer can take hold unchecked and spread to other organs if left too long. This is when cancer becomes incurable, compared to being treatable if found early.

Thankfully, not all delays will have such an awful outcome. For example, if you've read my story, you'll have read about Mags in chapter 1, the lady who gave me the best hug in the world. She had put off her routine mammogram three months earlier because she just didn't want to go to her mammogram appointment. After I was diagnosed, she decided to reschedule, and by a strange quirk of fate, Mags was diagnosed with breast cancer. Thankfully it was treatable, and, after surgery and radiotherapy, she made a full recovery. If there's one thing, I can thank my diagnosis for, it's that it prompted Mags to get checked.

I'm not suggesting a delay of a few hours or even a few weeks will make a difference to your diagnosis and prognosis – it probably won't – but what you don't want are delays that stretch into months because this is when potentially irreversible damage may occur.

What Are The Signs Of Breast Cancer?

Although you probably already know how breast cancer can present itself, it's worth reminding that breast cancer isn't always a lump. There are a few signs you need to be aware of. One of my good friends, Dawn-Marie Wilson, who unfortunately is no longer with us, was instrumental in the "Know your Lemons" campaign run by the Know Your Lemons Foundation. With their kind permission, I'm replicating their diagram, because it illustrates really well, what we should be looking for.

Learn the 12 signs of breast cancer:

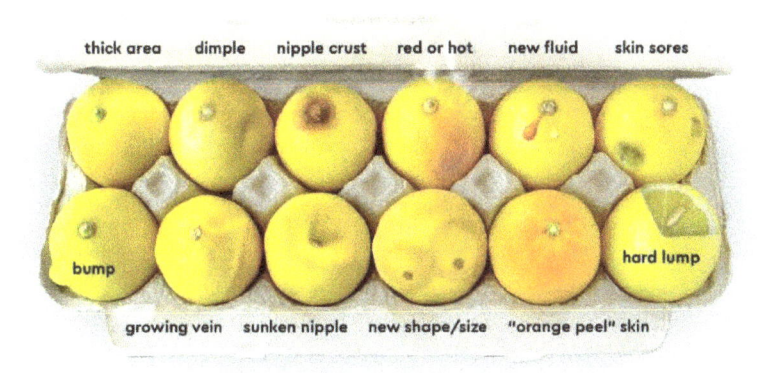

thick area | dimple | nipple crust | red or hot | new fluid | skin sores
bump | growing vein | sunken nipple | new shape/size | "orange peel" skin | hard lump

knowyourlemons.org/app

KNOW YOUR LEMONS APP

As you can see from the diagram, some of the signs are surprising – however, if you find one of these, it doesn't automatically mean cancer, but it strongly indicates that you should go to your doctor as soon as you can.

Once you've seen your doctor, they may be able to diagnose you quite easily with something far less worrying than cancer, but equally, if they are not sure, the normal process is to refer you to be seen by a specialist breast clinic.

Around 80% of referrals to a breast clinic result in a condition that is easily treated such as a cyst, a fatty or hormonal lump, an infection etc. So, although it can be daunting, please go. The clinic will aim to see you quickly, usually within two weeks (a month maximum) of the referral.

What Happens At A Breast Clinic?

At your appointment you may have several tests, and this really depends on the clinic, but these can include:

- a. A mammogram.
- b. An ultrasound.
- c. A biopsy of the area (if something needs investigating further).
- d. Inserting a "marker" into the affected area (again for further investigating).
- e. A meeting with a breast doctor or nurse – either during one of the tests or accompanying one of the scans

f. You may also be referred for one or more of the following scans:
- MRI (either breast, torso, or full body)
- CT (either a specific area or full body)
- Bone scan

All these tests are bearable – the mammogram can be a bit painful as it squashes your breast tissue between two plates, but it's over in a minute or two, so a few deep breaths should see you through that. The ultrasound is usually not a problem. If you've ever been pregnant, it's the same thing. There will be some pushing down on the breast tissue, and the worst bit is probably the cold gel they put on your breast but again, it's over very quickly.

If something is seen on a mammogram or ultrasound, to be sure what it is, you will probably have a biopsy taken and/or a marker inserted. Taking a biopsy and inserting a marker is a little painful, so you may be given a local anaesthetic. If I had to liken it to anything, it's a bit like getting your ear pierced with a piercing gun. You feel a slight crunch and hear the noise of a stapler. It's very quick (just like having your ears pierced), but it can cause a bruise for a few weeks. The biopsy stage of the process is THE most important part of the process because it will give an absolute answer to what's going on in your body. It can tell you if you have cancer or not and, if it's cancer, what type (this is explained later in the book). Without a biopsy, it's a bit like working in the dark so this is an essential part of the diagnosis process. Please don't forget, even though a biopsy is taken, it doesn't automatically mean it's cancer.

Further scans are not always needed but typically, they are requested if something shows on your breast and, if the nodes in your armpit look suspicious (there's more on this later in the book). If there's a suspicion of breast cancer in both areas, it is normal to have a scan just to double check that the cancer hasn't spread outside the breast. This can be overwhelmingly worrying, but please bear in mind this is routine.

Also, it's common for a scan to throw up something called a false positive. This can be when something shows that might be normal for you but abnormal for another – usually just your normal makeup and nothing sinister - and it can also be something temporary such as inflammation. Unfortunately, just to add to your stress levels, once noted, these will need investigating. The thing to bear in mind, is that these are all routine and, in most cases, won't reveal anything further. However, the anxiety it causes can make it difficult at a very worrying time.

After all tests are carried out, it's very normal for there to be a gap of around a week or two before you're called back for results. In exceptional circumstances, you may have results the same day, but this is rare. My view of cancer was "get it out and get it out quickly", so to be left waiting seemed awful. The reality is that the laboratory needs to carry out tests on your biopsy, and this can take time. Try not to worry, (easy to say I know), but this delay is fine, and won't harm your diagnosis or change your prognosis. In fact, it's more important that the diagnosis is correct, so you get the right treatment.

I Have Triple Negative Breast Cancer – What Now?

Once the results are in, if you have breast cancer, you'll be called to meet with a general doctor who will assign you an oncologist (a consultant who specialises in treating breast cancer), and surgeon (normally a consultant oncoplastic surgeon who specialises in breast cancer surgery).

You will either meet with the oncologist OR surgeon first – not see them both. It's not random. It very much depends on your diagnosis, and whether it's felt you will have surgery, or chemotherapy, first. Sometimes, the decision has already been made if your case has been put in front of a Multidisciplinary Team (MDT).

At every hospital, there's an MDT meeting each week attended by breast teams – oncologists, surgeons, radiographers, laboratory staff and usually breast care nurses. Each case, newly diagnosed, is discussed and a rough plan of action is decided, and consultants are appointed. This is a very basic description of what happens, but it does mean that there have been lots of input to your initial care already – not just one brain!

If you have a complex diagnosis – perhaps your laboratory results are showing you have an unusual type of cancer - more tests might be required, and your case may be assigned to the consultant who has the most knowledge in that area. Just as an aside, MDT meetings happen weekly, and if there are any changes to your diagnosis or treatment at any point, these will be discussed at the next meeting.

It might be useful to show you a graph of a "typical" diagnosis and treatment timeline, BUT please bear in mind, each hospital has their own timeframes, and ways of doing things, but generally speaking you'll probably follow this, or a similar pattern.

Expect that delays may happen along the way. For example, if you don't heal well after surgery, or have a complication, everything stops until you're better. Delays in treatment can happen at any time, and can be very scary but the majority of cancer patients have at least one delay of a few weeks at some point. Sometimes you can have multiple delays. Do not be alarmed if this happens. Delays are for a good reason, and you need to be as well as you can be when having chemotherapy etc.

Typical Timeline for Diagnosis and Treatment

Potential Steps & Timeframe from Diagnosis to end of Treatment

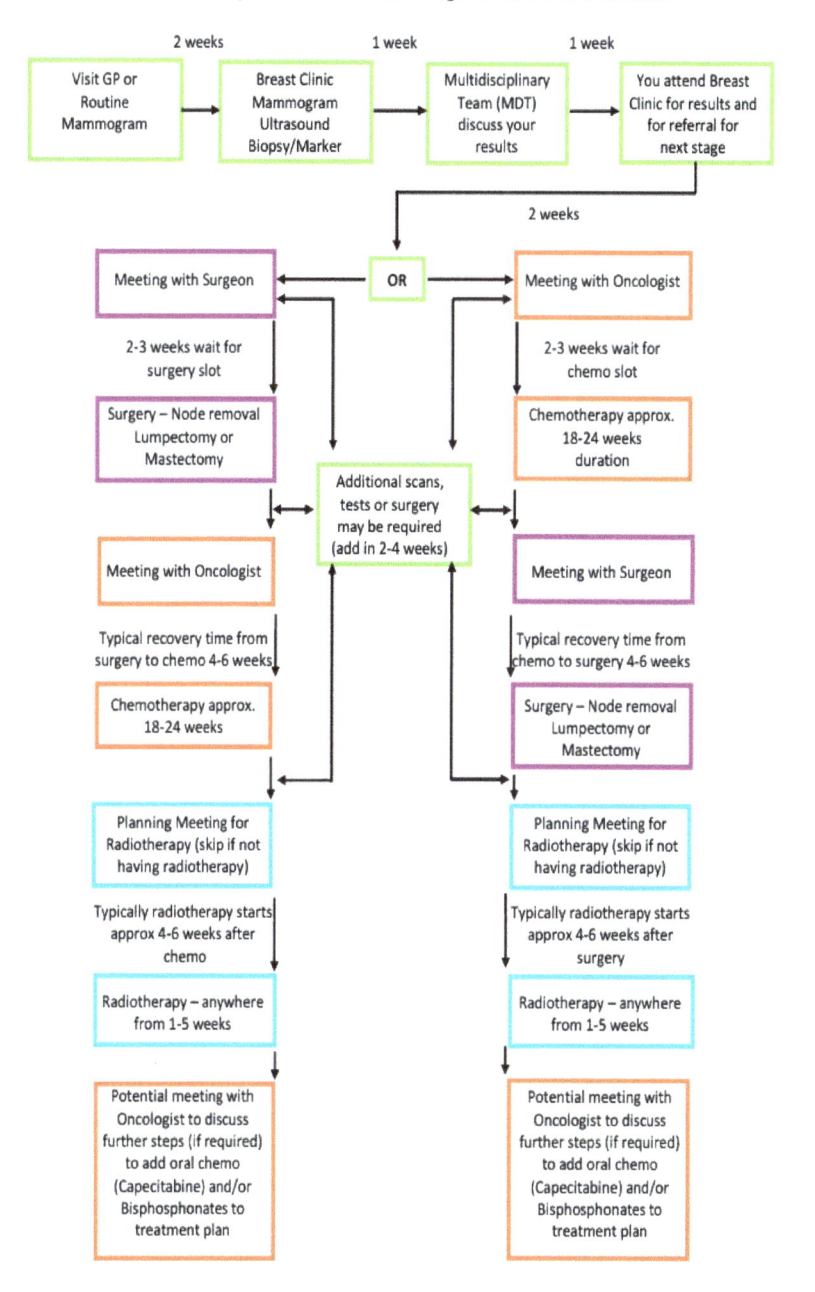

```
[Visit GP or Routine Mammogram] --2 weeks--> [Breast Clinic Mammogram Ultrasound Biopsy/Marker] --1 week--> [Multidisciplinary Team (MDT) discuss your results] --1 week--> [You attend Breast Clinic for results and for referral for next stage]
```

↓ 2 weeks

[Meeting with Surgeon] ← **OR** → [Meeting with Oncologist]

- 2-3 weeks wait for surgery slot
- 2-3 weeks wait for chemo slot

[Surgery – Node removal Lumpectomy or Mastectomy] [Chemotherapy approx. 18-24 weeks duration]

[Additional scans, tests or surgery may be required (add in 2-4 weeks)]

[Meeting with Oncologist] [Meeting with Surgeon]

- Typical recovery time from surgery to chemo 4-6 weeks
- Typical recovery time from chemo to surgery 4-6 weeks

[Chemotherapy approx. 18-24 weeks] [Surgery – Node removal Lumpectomy or Mastectomy]

[Planning Meeting for Radiotherapy (skip if not having radiotherapy)] [Planning Meeting for Radiotherapy (skip if not having radiotherapy)]

- Typically radiotherapy starts approx 4-6 weeks after chemo
- Typically radiotherapy starts approx 4-6 weeks after surgery

[Radiotherapy – anywhere from 1-5 weeks] [Radiotherapy – anywhere from 1-5 weeks]

[Potential meeting with Oncologist to discuss further steps (if required) to add oral chemo (Capecitabine) and/or Bisphosphonates to treatment plan] [Potential meeting with Oncologist to discuss further steps (if required) to add oral chemo (Capecitabine) and/or Bisphosphonates to treatment plan]

CHAPTER 3

UNDERSTANDING BREAST CANCER

What is Breast Cancer? - The Scientific Bit

At diagnosis, you will probably be worried that you've done something to start the cancer. You haven't! Let's explore this a bit more.

Breast cancer is, unfortunately, the most common cancer in the UK and not only affects women but men too. Breast cancer starts when cells begin to grow in an abnormal and uncontrolled way causing cancer to form as a tumour. There isn't a "one size fits all" that will tell you exactly why this has happened, but there are certain known risk factors, described later. Understanding how cancer starts may be helpful because it can be really confusing how, one minute you can be fine, and the next you have cancer. Let's explore this further.

Cancer starts with our genes, DNA, and how cells grow and change. Our bodies are made up of cells, and inside the cells are strings of DNA. These are individual to you. Unbelievably, in every cell, there are around 2 meters of DNA. The DNA is the brain that tells cells what to do. If you were to look at a "string" of DNA, you would see it's made up of genes. Each human being will have around 25,000 genes in total.

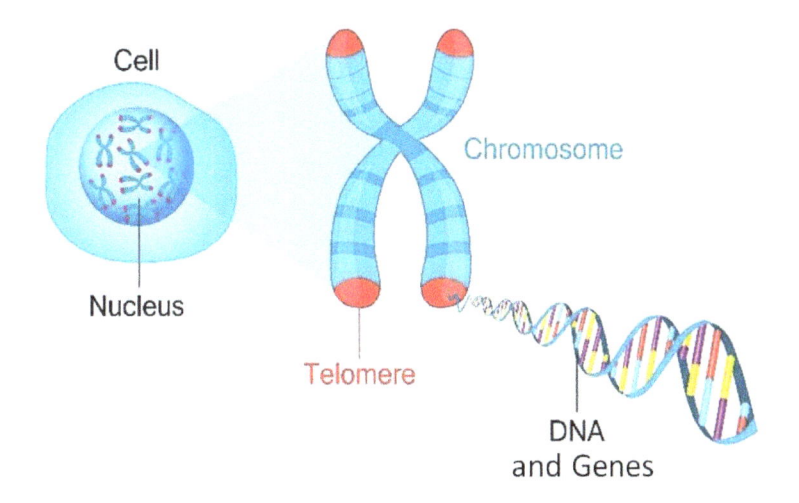

Cell — Nucleus — Chromosome — Telomere — DNA and Genes

We are all individuals because 50% of our DNA comes from our father, and 50% from our mother. The genes make "you". So, for example, genes are responsible for your eye, hair, skin colour, how you grow and reproduce, how you behave etc. Family members will share similar DNA, but when your genes combine, they will do so in a way that's individual to you.

Some genes specifically control how a cell will grow and divide and this is where cancer comes in. Cells divide all the time throughout our life, and sometimes, a fault or mistake occurs. The fault can happen at any time, and there's no way to predict when this may happen. Your body can motor on for years cancer free, cells dividing and multiplying happily, and then suddenly, a cell develops a fault. This may be due to an inherited faulty gene that previously your body has ignored, but equally, our bodies are machines, and unfortunately, it can just be unlucky that we have a mechanical blip, and our cells develop a fault.

When a fault occurs, our body sometimes detect it and will repair the cells – if the cells can't be repaired, they may even self-destruct! Our immune system may also recognise an "invader" and that too might jump in and kill the cell. Our bodies are truly amazing, aren't they? Who knew we had Star Wars going on all the time!?

So, if we have so many defence systems, how can cancer survive? Cancer begins when our body fail to recognise, or fails to kill, the cells that will be harmful to us. The faulty cells then start to multiply and don't perform as they would normally. They misunderstand what their genes should be telling them to do. It's a bit like when we ask our partners to take the bins out and they don't hear us! Not all cells that develop faults will cause cancer, but in important genes, they can.

What do I mean by "important genes"? There are 4 types of gene that are specifically linked to how a cell, develops, divides, and grows and it's when a change occurs in one of them that faults appear, and cancer takes hold. Although you don't need to know much more about this, it's interesting as a starting point should you want to read how drugs are being developed, because they often target these areas. These 4 genes are:

1. Genes that repair other damaged genes (DNA repair genes)

2. Genes that encourage cells to multiply (oncogenes)

3. Genes that stop the cell multiplying (tumour suppressor genes)

4. Genes that tell a cell to die (self-destruction genes)

So, if we look at a cell that has developed a fault and hasn't self-destructed, why doesn't our immune system shut it down? Actually, in many cases, the immune system WILL "see" the defective misshapen cells, jump into action and kill them, but sometimes cancer cells develop and find a way to "hide" from our immune system. Our immune system is then blind, can't see the cells, and the rogue cells are left to grow into cancerous tumours. If you're interested to read about our immune system, and how drugs called "immunotherapy" have been used to turn our immune system back on to help beat cancer, there's a chapter further in the book.

What Causes Breast Cancer?

So, we've looked at how a cancer may start, but what does that mean for you? How may it have started for you, and what are the risk factors?

Around 5-10% of breast cancers are caused by an inherited defective gene, where typically, there will be a family history of breast or ovarian cancer. You either have a defective gene or you don't – this is something you will be born with. The main genes identified for an increased risk of breast (and ovarian) cancer are called "BRCA genes", BRCA1 and BRCA2 (pronounced Bracca - BRCA stands for BReast CAncer). However, there are other genes such as PALB2, ATM, CHEK2, and quite a few more that are associated with an increased risk of breast cancer. There are also other genes being identified all the time (please see the chapter on genetic testing). It's also important to say that we all have the BRCA, PALB2 genes etc., but if they don't contain an inherited defect, they are not a risk to us.

But what if you don't have a defective gene? How can cancer start? It's easy to think you may have done something to cause cancer, but there's no concrete evidence to say that's correct – in fact, you may just be unlucky. As you read earlier, I mentioned it could come down to a temporary manufacturing defect, however, there are known risk factors for developing a breast cancer, which are, in order of risk, as follows:

- Being female.
- Getting older – as depressing as this is, the older you get, the more your risk increases. Increasing age means more defects accumulate so there is an increased risk of developing a cancer i.e., the manufacturing blip.
- Being overweight or leading a sedentary lifestyle.
- Your reproductive history (if you're female) – Starting periods early in life (before the age of 12) and/or starting menopause after the age of 55 exposes women to hormones for a longer period

of time, raising the risk of breast cancer. IVF, HRT, and contraception where certain hormones are used also fall into this category, as does extreme levels of stress. These changes are classed as hormonal, and you can read more about this later in the book.

- Previous radiation therapy.

- Dense breast tissue – ladies with denser breast tissue have a higher risk of developing breast cancer.

- As mentioned earlier, family history of breast or ovarian cancer. Having a faulty gene means you have a higher risk of developing breast cancer. In some cases, up to 80% higher, than somebody without a defective gene, but you can see the risk is much lower than, for example, age.

- Environmental factors are less clear cut and not a strong risk factor for breast cancers, but they might include sun damage or exposure to chemicals. Smoking, and the use of sunbeds, would fall into this category as well.

This list is not exhaustive but gives you an overview. You may be able to identify with some, or none, but rather than torture yourself with "what ifs", it's better to look forward at how to treat, and get yourself, cancer-free.

Cancer hits people who are old, young, fit, unfit, eat healthily, eat unhealthily and of all ethnic origins. I know lots of ladies who, after diagnosis and treatment, changed nothing in their lives and are still happily clear of cancer. Others have changed their diet, lifestyle, cut back or made radical changes and have had a recurrence (i.e., another breast cancer). If you want to cut out things in your diet that's great. If you want to get fit – that's great too. You must do what you feel is right for you.

For now, however, let's stop there, otherwise, it will become too technical. To sum up, it's highly unlikely you haven't done anything to start your cancer, so put that thought to the back of your mind.

Let's look a bit more closely at what you may be told about your cancer at diagnosis and try to demystify some of the terminology.

CHAPTER 4

UNDERSTANDING THE BASICS OF YOUR BREAST CANCER

Before being diagnosed, I just thought breast cancer was breast cancer. I had no idea it could grow in different parts of the breast, that there were different types, sub-types, and special types. That was a complete shock and a very steep learning curve!

A basic understanding will help with your diagnosis and give you a better idea of your individual diagnosis, what's happening and why, but you don't need to know any of it if you don't want to. Many, many, many people diagnosed with breast cancer, will not want to know the details, and that's perfectly fine. There's no right or wrong way – there's just your way! For others, they need to know what they have, and it might give them back a bit of control. So, if you want to know a bit more, I've broken it down as simply as possible into sections. Each of these sections are expanded further on, but the overview is as follows:

- The **exact place** in your breast that cancer has been identified. This is important because you can have areas of cancer and pre-cancerous growths and they usually appear in different parts of the breast.

- **Stage** of breast cancer (this means the size of the cancer tumour(s), and whether there are any affected nodes in your armpit or spread to other parts of the body). An easy way to remember Stage is that the **S** of **S**tage means **Size** and/or **Spread**. Staging is explained fully later.

- **Grade** of breast cancer (this means how quickly the cancer cells are growing). An easy way to remember this is the **G** of **Grade** can stand for **Growth**. The grades of breast cancer are explained further in the book.

- **Type** of breast cancer and receptor status. Again, all explained later.

The information about your personal cancer, will be gleaned from biopsies and scans, and they are key to determining your individual diagnosis and treatment. Unfortunately, there is normally a wait of up to 2 weeks after those tests/scans, because your results need to be combined, and then the oncologist or surgeon will put together your individual treatment plan.

Where is Breast Cancer or Changes found in your Breast?

Let's look first at where cancer may be in your breast, as this is probably the first thing you'll be told.

There are two main areas in the breast structure that may be flagged for further investigation (1) The first area is within the breast tissue or skin where cancer cells have "invaded" normal healthy tissue. This is called an "invasive ductal carcinoma" and the area that will be treated as it's always classified as cancer (you can see this on the right side of the graph) (2) The second area is of less concern because it's classed as pre-cancerous, which means there are changes to normal cells that may, or may not, become cancer. These cells are contained in the ducts or glands, which is why you'll see it referred to as "ductal carcinoma in situ" (this is shown in the middle portion of the graph). As you'll see later, it's not uncommon to have both types. As you read on, you may want to refer to this diagram and the terminology:

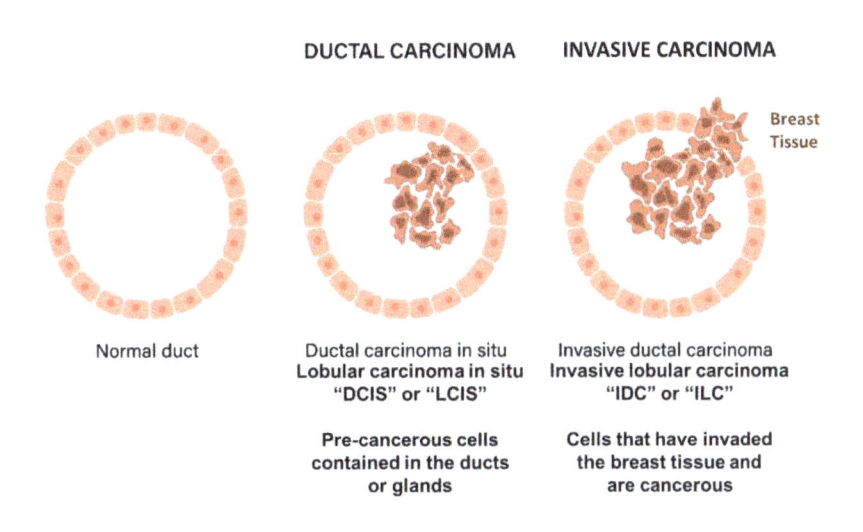

DUCTAL CARCINOMA   **INVASIVE CARCINOMA**

Breast Tissue

Normal duct

Ductal carcinoma in situ
Lobular carcinoma in situ
"DCIS" or "LCIS"

Pre-cancerous cells contained in the ducts or glands

Invasive ductal carcinoma
Invasive lobular carcinoma
"IDC" or "ILC"

Cells that have invaded the breast tissue and are cancerous

Let's look at invasive breast cancer first because if you're reading this book, it's likely that's what you've been diagnosed with – so we will start from the right and work to the middle.

Explaining Invasive Breast Cancer

Within the umbrella term of "invasive" breast cancer, there are two different types. The most common is Invasive

Ductal Cancer (IDC), and the less common, Invasive Lobular Carcinoma (ILC). You can see both on the right-hand side of the diagram where the cells have broken out of the duct into the breast tissue and become "invaders". IDC is normally always cancer but IDC and ILC are a little different. The chances are, you will have an IDC, but I'm outlining both below.

So, what's the difference between IDC and ILC if they're both invaders and both cancer?

Invasive Ductal Cancer (IDC)

Up to 80% of Triple Negative breast cancers will have the label "invasive ductal carcinoma" (**IDC**). IDC is the most common type of breast cancer identified and, when contained in the breast and/or nodes and nowhere else in the body, it's called "early" or "primary" breast cancer. An invasive breast cancer has probably started in one of the ducts in the breast and then spread (or invaded), into the breast tissue and surrounding areas. Once it has invaded or infiltrated the breast tissue, it has the potential to spread out of the breast which is why correct diagnosis and treatment is essential. As mentioned above, the majority of Triple Negative breast cancers will fall under the umbrella of IDC, and you may see this in your notes and copy letters.

Invasive Lobular Carcinoma (ILC)

In around 5-10% of breast cancers, a less common form of invasive cancer is found, and it's called Invasive Lobular

Carcinoma (ILC). If you are diagnosed with "lobular cancer" you need to pay attention to whether it's in the glands OR if it's invasive only because, confusingly, "lobular" is in both names. It's important to understand the difference because, in the glands it's not cancerous, invasive it is.

Simply, a lobular cancer refers to how it looks under the microscope and that's typically a lump. It can react differently to IDC in that, if it's invasive, there may be a few areas found of invasive tumours. Lobular breast cancer is more prevalent in older women (although younger people can be affected). The good news is that it does have an encouraging prognosis.

Pre-cancerous Cells

I am not going to be focussing on the middle section of the graph, Ductal Carcinoma In Situ (DCIS), as it's not actually cancer, so a full explanation is in the next section only. However, it may be helpful to refer to, if at any point you are diagnosed with DCIS because it can often be found sitting next to an invasive cancer.

Ductal Carcinoma in Situ (DCIS)

Pre-cancerous cells can be found in the ducts or glands of the breast. However, calling it "pre-cancerous" is a bit misleading because, in many cases, it will never become cancer. IF DCIS is going to become cancerous, it will break out of the ducts or glands into the surrounding breast tissue and will become "invasive" but this may never happen.

Quite often, DCIS is detected sitting near, or next to, an invasive breast cancer, and can be an incidental finding as it doesn't always show on scans. DCIS can happily sit in your ducts or glands for years without doing anything but, as it may become cancerous, when identified, it is usually removed at the same time as the invasive tumour. If you only have DCIS, it may be treated, or it may be left alone.

DCIS might be larger in size than the invasive tumour. For example, you could have a 10cm area of DCIS, but your invasive tumour is only 1cm. Your oncologist/surgeon's focus will be on the 1cm because that's the bit that's cancer. So, when the size (and staging) of your cancer is discussed, you'll find that the DCIS isn't included, and is mostly ignored. Using this example, your area of cancer would be 1cm.

Once found, DCIS is analysed to detect whether it's slow or fast growing, and it will be given a grade - low, medium, or high grade. If your DCIS is a high grade, there is a strong possibility that the cells will become cancerous within 5 years and will leach into your breast tissue, to become an invasive tumour. Low or medium grade DCIS are slower growing and less likely to develop into an invasive cancer, (still possible though).

Lobular Carcinoma In Situ (LCIS)

Another form of changed cells, similar to DCIS, is called Lobular Carcinoma In Situ (LCIS), and is found in the breast lobules (glands that specifically make milk). The abnormal cells are all contained within the inner lining of the lobules.

While DCIS is considered a pre-cancer, it is unclear whether LCIS is definitely a pre-cancer or, if it is just a general risk factor for developing breast cancer. LCIS rarely seems to become an invasive cancer, but it does raise the risk of getting breast cancer in either breast. It will generally not need removing but may lead to a recommendation for breast screening on an annual basis, rather than the typical three-yearly. LCIS increases your risk of developing breast cancer, in either breast, for at least ten years after diagnosis

Analysing DCIS/LCIS

An important part, when reviewing DCIS, is, not only to look at the grade but to look at the cell structure as it may give your oncologist a heads-up as to how the DCIS may, or may not, grow. The biopsy analysis of DCIS will also include its "type" (see below for more information). Sometimes the DCIS doesn't have any live cells – our bodies have already killed it off, or it could have patches that are dead and other areas still active.

A laboratory may report on what the cells of your DCIS look like. The cell structure and shape can be broken down into Solid/Comedo, Cribriform, Micropapillary, Papillary, and Pleomorphic. It's useful for oncologists to know, but of no benefit for patients other than just to know! So, for example, mine was "solid" which means the cells completely filled the duct. Sometimes labs call this Comedo which means "plugged". Cribriform cells have gaps between them - a bit like Swiss cheese. Micropapillary, Papillary and Pleomorphic cells are shaped like ferns - they have branches that reach out, and these are more likely to reach beyond the ducts, and into the breast tissue where it becomes invasive.

How does Breast Cancer spread to other areas?

As well as looking at your breast, your team will look at your "nodes" which extend from your armpit outwards. Even if your cancer has spread from the breast to the nodes, this is still an early or primary breast cancer, but investigating the nodes is essential because once cancer gets into the nodes, it has a pathway out of the breast, and into your body. Before you panic, it's the job of the nodes to catch and keep the cancer cells without allowing them to move anywhere else, and in most cases that's exactly what they do. So, let's look at this is more detail.

Sentinel and Axillary Nodes

In our breasts (and actually all around our body), we have a filtration system made up of a network of "nodes". This is called the lymphatic system and in very basic terms, it's a defence system, aimed at catching invaders and neutralising them. In this case, cancer cells.

In the breast, this network is made up of "sentinel nodes" (and in the diagram over the page, the first ones in the chain). which are our first line of defence. Behind them, there are axillary nodes that deal with anything that's slipped past or overwhelmed the sentinels. The number of nodes we have in our body is completely individual to us. In the armpit, there can be anything from 8 to 50!

If the nodes have been overwhelmed and cancer cells get past them all, they can reach other parts of your body and organs.

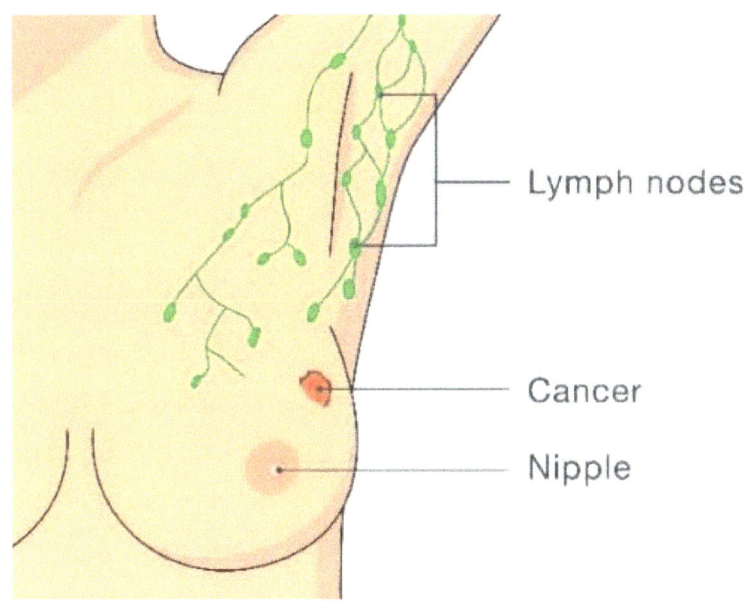

Very confusingly, if you have cancer in your nodes, this is technically called metastatic cancer, but the term metastatic is usually only used in the main for Stage 4 cancers, where the cancer has spread to other organs around the body. When used in conjunction with discussing nodes, it literally means that the cells have left the immediate breast area and travelled to the nodes - so please don't be worried if you see this term associated with your nodes. It means a **localised spread** NOT a spread to other parts of the body.

Although it's thought that having "positive" lymph nodes may increase your risk of cancer leaving the breast area, I've seen ladies with 30 affected nodes who are into double figures past treatment with no recurrence or spread. Similarly, I've seen ladies with no node involvement, have spread. So, whilst the presence of having positive nodes is important, and a factor in your treatment, it doesn't necessarily predict an outcome.

There is another way known that cancer can spread around the body and that's called:

Lymphovascular Invasion (LVI)

Confusingly, because this has "lymph" in its title, people assume that it refers to the lymph nodes mentioned above. It doesn't. It refers to the lymphatic system that carries blood around your body, to and from your breast, using lymphatic channels and blood vessels. So, if cancer cells break into the blood carrying channels, they have the potential to spread to the rest of the body.

However, as with the nodes, a positive lymphovascular invasion (LVI), is not a definitive indicator of poor prognosis. LVI can be a pre-cursor to cells moving from the tumour to the nodes, so it doesn't necessarily indicate that the cells will be found elsewhere in the body. LVI is NOT part of the staging process. So, if you have it, you will still be classed as having an early or primary breast cancer.

CHAPTER 5

STAGES OF BREAST CANCER

A "stage" in breast cancer gives an indication of the size and spread, i.e., how big, or small, your tumour is, if nodes have been affected, and whether cancer has spread to other organs. Remember that "**s**tage" means **s**ize/**s**pread. Although it's a "nice to know" and understand, it's more of a common language for medical professionals to discuss diagnosis on the same level playing field. It's also useful for cancer patients when chatting to others.

It is important to note that, unlike other parts of your diagnosis, staging can change. For example, if your tumour was measured at 1.5cm on a scan but at surgery was 3cm, it may result in your staging changing. This is very common and nothing to worry about.

Whilst this book is predominately for those diagnosed with stages 1-3 (i.e., an early or primary breast cancer), classed as "treatable" <u>and</u> "curable", the following will describe staging as it relates to Stage 0, 1, 2, 3, and Stage 4.

One thing to bear in mind is that you shouldn't be worried whether you're stage 1, 2 or 3. The treatment is normally the same and the size of tumour does not mean a worse prognosis. Size really doesn't matter! The size of a tumour does not indicate how aggressive it is. You can have a slow-growing, huge tumour that is just hanging around not doing much, but then you can have a tiny cancer that's growing and multiplying at the speed of light and the school bully!

There are two methods to stage cancer. Some cancer teams will use a numerical system (i.e., stage 0 to 4), but others will use a lettering system (TNM) and sometimes, a combination of both. Due to the complexity of explaining what Staging is, I am replicating information published by Cancer Research UK (with their kind permission).

Since giving their permission, Cancer Research has published a simplified version of the numerical system, but I am replicating the older version as it has more information. Cancer Research UK's latest published advice on staging can be viewed at www.cancerresearchuk.org.

If you haven't been told your stage, you'll be able to work it out from the following as lots of ladies are not told their stage:

STAGES OF BREAST CANCER

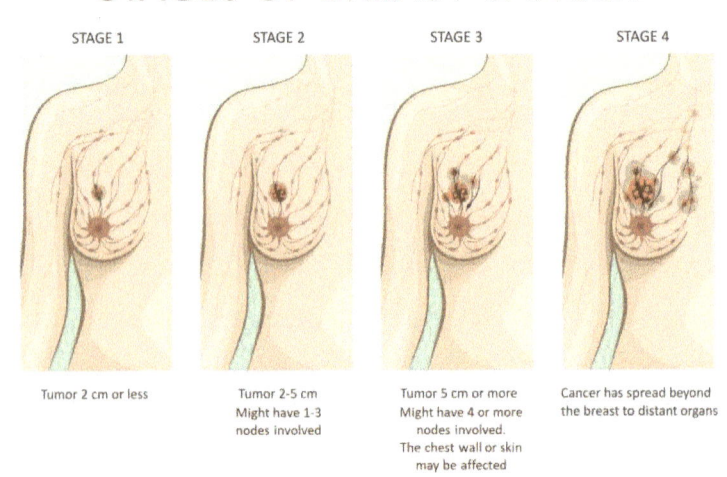

STAGE 1
Tumor 2 cm or less

STAGE 2
Tumor 2-5 cm
Might have 1-3 nodes involved

STAGE 3
Tumor 5 cm or more
Might have 4 or more nodes involved.
The chest wall or skin may be affected

STAGE 4
Cancer has spread beyond the breast to distant organs

Stage 0

You'll notice that Stage 0 is not included in the graph above – this is because, as mentioned earlier it's not classed as cancer. Stage 0 is used to describe pre-cancerous changes that may or may not become cancer. If you remember from the previous chapter, DCIS and LCIS (i.e., pre-cancerous cells contained in a duct, gland etc) would be classed as Stage 0.

Stage 1

Stage 1 breast cancer means that the cancer is small and only in the breast tissue, or it might be found in lymph nodes close to the breast. It is an early-stage breast cancer. Stage 1 breast cancer has two groups:

Stage 1A means that the tumour is 2 centimetres (cm) or smaller and has not spread outside the breast

Stage 1B means that small areas of breast cancer cells are found in the lymph nodes close to the breast and that:

- no tumour is found in the breast

or

- the breast tumour is 2cm or smaller

Stage 2

Stage 2 breast cancer means that the cancer is either in the breast or in the nearby lymph nodes or both. It is early-stage breast cancer. Stage 2 breast cancer has two groups: stage 2A and 2B.

Stage 2A means <u>one</u> of the following

- there is no tumour or a tumour 2 centimetres (cm) or smaller in the breast and cancer cells are found in 1 to 3 lymph nodes in the armpit or in the lymph nodes near the breastbone

- the tumour is larger than 2cm but not larger than 5cm and there is no cancer in the lymph nodes

- Stage 2B means one of the following

- the tumour is larger than 2cm but not larger than 5cm and there are small areas of cancer cells in the lymph nodes

- the tumour is larger than 2cm but not larger than 5cm and the cancer has spread to 1 to 3 lymph nodes in the armpit or to the lymph nodes near the breastbone

- the tumour is larger than 5cm and hasn't spread to the lymph nodes

Stage 3

Stage 3 means that cancer has spread from the breast to lymph nodes close to the breast or to the skin of the breast or to the chest wall. It is also called locally advanced breast cancer. Stage 3 breast cancer is divided into three groups.

Stage 3A means one of the following:

- no tumour is seen in the breast, or the tumour may be any size and cancer is found in 4 to 9 lymph glands under the arm or in the lymph glands near the breastbone
- the tumour is larger than 5cm and small clusters of breast cancer cells are in the lymph nodes
- the tumour is more than 5cm and has spread into up to 3 lymph nodes in the armpit or to the lymph nodes near the breastbone

Stage 3B means the tumour has spread to the skin of the breast or the chest wall. The chest wall means the structures surrounding and protecting the lungs, such as the ribs, muscles, skin, or connective tissues. Cancer has made the skin break down (an ulcer) or caused swelling. Cancer may have spread to up to 9 lymph nodes in the armpit or to the lymph nodes near the breastbone. Cancer that has spread to the skin of the breast might be an inflammatory breast cancer.

Stage 3C means the tumour can be any size, or there may be no tumour. But there is cancer in the skin of the breast, causing swelling or an ulcer and it has spread to the chest wall. It has also spread to one or more of the following structures:

- 10 or more lymph nodes in the armpit
- lymph nodes above or below the collar bone
- lymph nodes in the armpit and near the breastbone

For treatment, doctors divide stage 3C breast cancer into cancers that can be operated on (operable breast cancers) and those that can't (inoperable cancer).

Stage 4

Stage 4 breast cancer means that cancer has spread to other parts of the body. It is also called advanced cancer, secondary breast cancer, or metastatic breast cancer.

In stage 4 breast cancer:

- the tumour can be any size

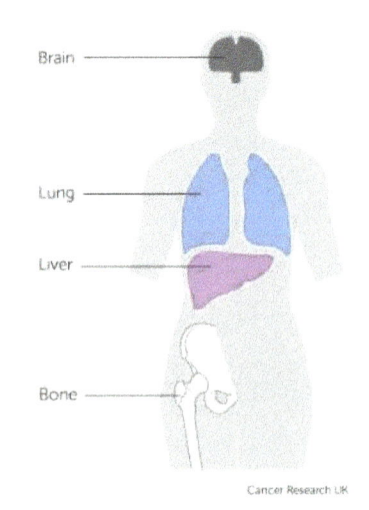

- the lymph nodes may or may not contain cancer cells

- cancer has spread (metastasised) to other parts of the body such as the bones, lungs, liver, or brain

It may be helpful to explain stage 4 in a little more detail - When cancer spreads beyond the breast it's more challenging and usually means that life may be limited. There are people I've known who have been classed as cancer free (or NED – no evidence of disease) following a stage 4 diagnosis, but this isn't common. It really depends on where cancer has spread, the extent of the cancer, and if it can be surgically removed or not (and, of course, how well it responds to treatment). With stage 4, there is always the possibility that the cancer will come back in the same place or elsewhere, so for many stage 4 patients, treatment is ongoing.

TNM staging

This alternative type of staging is becoming more popular as it's easier for oncologists to compare.

TNM stands for Tumour, Node, Metastasis. Your scans and tests give some information about the stage of cancer, but, as with the other system mentioned above, your doctor might not be able to tell you the exact stage until you have surgery. Again, with the kind permission of Cancer Research UK I am replicating their wording on the TNM staging system.

- T describes the size of the tumour.
- N describes whether there are any cancer cells in the lymph nodes.
- M describes whether the cancer has spread to a different part of the body.

The system uses letters and numbers to describe the cancer.

- **T** refers to the size of the cancer and how far it has spread into nearby tissue – it can be 1, 2, 3 or 4, with 1 being small and 4 large.
- **N** refers to whether the cancer has spread to the lymph nodes – it can be between 0 (no lymph nodes

containing cancer cells) and 3 (lots of lymph nodes containing cancer cells).

- **M** refers to whether the cancer has spread to another part of the body – it can either be 0 (the cancer hasn't spread) or 1 (the cancer has spread).

So, for example, a small cancer that has spread to the lymph nodes but not to anywhere else in the body may be T2 N1 M0 (i.e., a tumour of around 2cm or more (T2), one node showing cancer (N1) but no spread to other parts of the body (M0)). Or a more advanced cancer that has spread may be T4 N3 M1 (i.e., a large tumour in the breast (T4), multiple node involvement (N3) and spread to other organs (M1)).

The letter c is sometimes used before the letters TNM. For example, cT2 N1, M0. This stands for the clinical stage. It means that the stage is based on what the doctor knows about the cancer <u>before</u> surgery. Doctors may look at your tests results and use the clinical information from examining you, but this may change after surgery/treatment.

The letter p is sometimes used before the letters TNM. For example, pT4. This stands for the pathological stage. It means that the staging is based on examining cancer cells in the lab <u>after</u> surgery and will be an exact diagnosis.

CHAPTER 6

GRADES OF BREAST CANCER

What does Grading mean?

Thankfully it's far easier to understand grading than stages! Grading is a system that tells your oncologist how fast, or slow, your cancer is growing, and what the cells look like. You may remember from an earlier chapter, an easy way to remember what grade means is by using the G in Grade to make the word Growth! There are 3 Grades:

- Grade 1 - These are the slowest growing cancer cells, and they're growing in a well organised format. Not many of them will be making new cancer cells.

- Grade 2 - These are growing faster than grade 1 and do not look like normal cells as they are beginning to look misshapen. They will be dividing more quickly.

- Grade 3 - These cells are messy looking, without an organised pattern. They are dividing very quickly to make new cancer cells. A grade 3 tumour will be growing faster than a Grade 2 or Grade 1 tumour.

Do not be alarmed if you are diagnosed with a Grade 3 cancer. Chemotherapy and radiotherapy actually target the faster growing cells very effectively. Most Triple Negative breast cancer is Grade 3, however; some are grade 2 or even Grade 1, but this is less usual.

Whilst we are looking at the speed of tumours, there is an additional test that laboratories sometimes carry out to refine the speed of growth even further. Grades 1, 2 and 3 are quite general, so taking this a step further, they can tell whether the speed is at the lower or higher end of Grade 3. This test looks at the "proliferation" of cells (i.e., how quickly the cells are growing and multiplying), and it's called Ki-67. In a grade 3 breast cancer, a Ki-67 result of less than 10% is considered low, 10-20% borderline, and high if more than 20%. With my tumour, my proliferation rate (Ki-67) was over 80%, so I often describe it as the Usain Bolt of breast cancers! There are other similar tests that laboratories carry out to measure the same thing but the most common is Ki-67.

CHAPTER 7

TYPES OF BREAST CANCER

We've looked at where a cancer can be found in the breast, the size, spread and how fast it may be growing, but now we need to understand what Triple Negative breast cancer is, and how it's different to other breast cancers. I am briefly including information on hormonal breast cancer as more than one tumour may be found in your breast (and they may not all be Triple Negative) or you may be borderline for a hormonal breast cancer.

Breast cancers fall into categories. Three are classed as hormonal breast cancers and the fourth is Triple Negative. So, what's the difference?

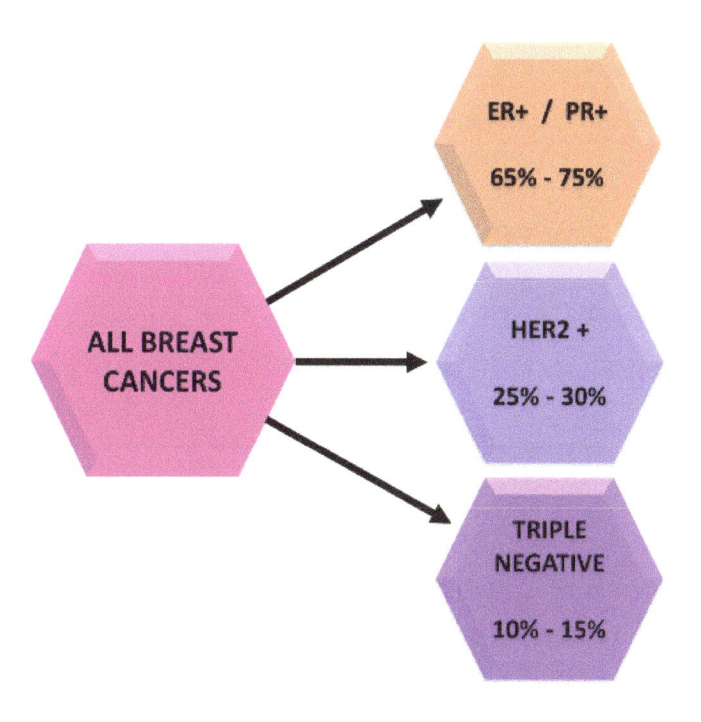

ALL BREAST CANCERS
- ER+ / PR+ 65% - 75%
- HER2 + 25% - 30%
- TRIPLE NEGATIVE 10% - 15%

Hormonal Breast Cancers (ER+, PR+ and HER2+)

If the tumour has positive receptors (a protein found on the cancer cell that triggers a growth reaction), it's called hormonal breast cancer. The cells will be fed by one (or more) hormones, namely, oestrogen (ER+), progesterone (PR+) or the snappily titled human epidermal growth factor receptor 2 – thankfully shortened to HER2- allowing them to grow! As you can see from the graph, ER+ and PR+ are the most common, accounting for 65-75% of all breast cancers. HER2+ is less common, making up 25-30% of all breast cancers.

So, what does that actually mean – what are positive receptors and why are they important? This is where the difference comes in between hormonal breast cancers and Triple Negative. As mentioned above, hormonal breast cancers are "fed" by hormones which allow the cancer to grow and spread. Scientists have found a way to turn off hormonal receptors, using targeted drugs, which cut off the food to the cancer cells, starving them, so they can't live in the body. So, once a hormonal breast cancer has been found and treated, these drugs can be taken to prevent another similar breast cancer from growing.

With Triple Negative breast cancer, there are no hormonal receptors and therefore, at the moment, there is nothing that can be taken to "turn off" what's allowing the cancer to grow. This is an area of much research, but for now, there isn't a targeted drug that can be taken to prevent a future Triple

Negative breast cancer from forming. Before you feel upset by that (and I'm sure you may be), read on.

The targeted drugs for hormonal breast cancers do have drawbacks though. If a patient with a hormonal breast cancer stops taking them, their cancer can come back at any time – even 10-25 years later. So, these preventative drugs have to be taken, usually, for the patient's lifetime. Also, because each drug targets a specific hormone, for example oestrogen, progesterone, HER2 etc, it won't stop a different type of breast cancer, or a Triple Negative cancer from starting. If a patient was taking an oestrogen targeted drug, they could still have a future HER2 or Triple Negative breast cancer. Having said that, the targeted therapies are essential in the war against hormonal breast cancer and do stop many new cancers forming.

Triple Negative Breast Cancer

If you are diagnosed with Triple Negative, your first thought may either be "negative – well that must be a good thing", OR you will hit the internet and then be thrown into a panic when you read words like "rare", "aggressive", and "more likely to return". I know it's easier said than done but try not to panic. Let's explore Triple Negative in a bit more detail.

As you can see from the graph, Triple Negative Breast Cancer accounts for around 10-15% of all breast cancers diagnosed, so it is often referred to as "rare", and this conjures up concerns that there will be less research, fewer resources etc. But, in reality, new treatments and drugs are being developed all the time, and there are also trials specifically for Triple Negative patients. So being rare doesn't mean you can't be treated, or they don't know how to – they do!

Now let's look at why it's considered to be fierce and aggressive – the two words you see most associated with Triple Negative. One of the reasons (as mentioned above) is there's no targeted drug that a Triple Negative patient can take after treatment has finished. In other words, nothing to prevent it from coming back. Patients often feel very alone after treatment has finished because there's no safety net.

Unfortunately, without this safety net, because of its aggressive nature, if a Triple Negative cancer is going to come back, it normally does so within the first one to three years after treatment ends. Each year after that, the risk lessens until at five to seven years, the risk is similar to that of somebody who has never had breast cancer. Whilst that sounds very worrying, if it does come back, it may still be within the breast or nodes and can be treated and cured once more. So, whilst the thought of having to go through treatment again is daunting, it can be done, and I have known several ladies who have had Triple Negative three times and are currently cancer free.

The aggressive nature of Triple Negative is probably what sets it apart from hormonal breast cancers. Being aggressive does have an advantage because chemotherapy was designed to kill off the fastest-growing misshapen cells, so typically, Triple Negative will respond well to chemotherapy.

Very occasionally, Triple Negative can become resistant to chemotherapy (just like antibiotics for an infection), and you may need to try several different ones before you hit the magic combination. For most diagnosed with Triple Negative, the chemotherapy regime will include a number of different chemotherapies, given at the same time, specifically for this reason. If chemotherapy doesn't work, immunotherapy might and, hopefully, that will be used more in the future for early-stage breast cancers.

Types in a Bit More Scientific Detail

Now we need to look a bit deeper to understand Triple Negative's reputation and what sets it apart from other breast cancers.

A tumour is normally made up of a population of cancer cells – sometimes they are all similar, and of one type, i.e., ER, PR, HER2 or Triple Negative so it's easy for your cancer to be given a classification or type. However, sometimes a tumour can contain multiple types of cells, for example it may have a combination of ER+ cells and Triple Negative cells etc., or any other combination.

If a tumour is made up of multiple cell types, some of the different populations may be killed off by our own defences as the tumour cells die, divide, or grow. So, for example, a tumour may start with more ER+ cells than anything else, but as it grows, the cells may lose their receptors and change to become Triple Negative until there's very little ER+ cells left. This can happen over a matter of weeks, so what started as, for example, an ER+ tumour, may well change to become a Triple Negative tumour.

Very occasionally, a tumour change may lead to a biopsy reporting incorrectly. A biopsy only takes a tiny portion of a tumour, and when a tumour changes, the changes may start in a few cells but then spread to others. If your biopsy hits the part that is changing OR hasn't started to change, you'll get different readings. This is quite rare, but it can happen, and it's why your diagnosis can change after surgery. This is rare, but it's worth mentioning especially when we look at HRT and hormones later in the book.

If that hasn't blown your mind – how about this ... If you have two separate tumours in the same breast, they may each have their own makeup! They're not always the same kind. For example, you could have one that is HER2+, and another that is Triple Negative! Typically, your oncologist will treat the more aggressive of the two because the same treatment is likely to work on both, so you'll be treated as if you were just Triple Negative.

Even more curious is that your tumour may be one type and your nodes another! This is far less common, but it can happen! It can also happen that a Triple Negative tumour changes to have hormonal receptors, although this is even rarer.

Just an aside, if your breast cancer has spread to other parts of your body, biopsies will be taken, if possible, to check what, if any, receptors may be found, and again, just because your main tumour may be one type, metastatic cancer may be different.

The only time that hormonal receptors are relevant for a Triple Negative patient is if their tumour has weakly positive readings for ER+, PR+ or HER2+. What that means is that most of the cancer cells will be Triple Negative but there's a small proportion that has hormonal receptors. In these instances, after the main treatment has finished for the Triple Negative cancer, your oncologist may offer the hormone targeted drugs mentioned above, to prevent a recurrence. Whilst the tablets should stop a future hormonal tumour, they are unlikely to ward off a future Triple Negative cancer, so you are normally given the choice of taking them or not. It's about weighing up the potential side effects against the risks. Each case will be different, but in most cases, patients try the tablets and if they feel well, they continue, but if they can't tolerate them, the oncologist will often advise stopping.

How do I know what type of Breast Cancer I have?

Your biopsy will be sent to a laboratory where tests are carried out and a pathology report sent to your consultant which will confirm whether you are positive or negative for each type. Various tests are used, and because each type reacts differently, the tumour is put through several specific tests. What this means is that on documentation, you may see a number after ER, PR and HER2 that will determine whether your tumour is positive for hormone receptors or negative. Unfortunately, ER and PR have one scoring system and HER2 another. This can cause confusion as the numbering ranges are different. Very briefly (and if you're Triple Negative you really don't need to know this), the scoring system is as follows:

ER / PR - Rated using the Allred Scale from 0 – 8:

0-2 = negative

3 = borderline/weakly positive.

4 and above = strongly positive and your cancer will be considered ER+ and/or PR+.

NB: If you have been diagnosed with Triple Negative but your ER/PR score is 3, this is when targeted drugs may be offered as described above, as a targeted therapy after treatment has finished.

HER2 - There are four commonly used tests, IHC, FISH, CISH and DDISH. IHC is normally the first test and scores from 0-3+

0 or 1+ means the breast cancer is HER2 **negative** (despite the + symbol)

2+ is borderline

3+ means the breast cancer is HER2 positive.

NB: If your tumour has a borderline result (i.e., 2+), the laboratory will carry out further tests to confirm a positive or negative HER2 diagnosis. It's highly unlikely you'll be given preventative tablets after treatment as this would mean you were positive for HER2+. However, if your tumour was TN and your nodes HER2+ for example, you may be given the choice of taking preventative medication.

Getting Technical – Special Types of Breast Cancer

I've outlined above the main types of breast cancer, hormonal, and Triple Negative, but laboratories will also analyse the cells that make up your tumour. Sometimes the cells will just look like normal cancer cells and will be described as "no special type" or NST. Around 70% of all hormonal positive and Triple Negative breast cancers are NST. This means that it's a bog-standard Triple Negative cancer without any unusual or rare makeup.

However, some cells may look very different and these fall into categories. Knowing the exact tumour make-up can help an oncologist predict how the cancer will grow or move around. These are still classed as Triple Negative tumours, but they are a "special type". Think of Triple Negative as the house but then a special type could be the doors and windows. It's still Triple Negative but the cells may grow and change in subtle ways. Treatment for these special types is usually the same as for a no special type Triple Negative but may have a different or preferred surgery option.

Let's look at the more common special types that may be associated with a Triple Negative tumour:

- **Inflammatory** – this can be difficult to diagnose as typically it presents as a reddening or change to the skin and can be confused with an infection. The cancer cells block the lymph channels, and this is what causes the changes to the skin, and it can (not always) be painful. It can also spread quite quickly, so typically with inflammatory, chemotherapy is given first and surgery options may be recommended strongly, one way rather than another.

- **Metaplastic** – Interestingly, Metaplastic wasn't defined as an actual special type of cancer on its own until around 1973, when the World Health Organisation recognised it as a sub-set breast cancer. Up until that point, it hadn't been recognised and this is probably because in terms of breast cancer, it's very rare. Only about 0.02%-5% of ALL breast cancers diagnosed are Metaplastic. With this type, there is a mixture of two different types of cells called mesenchymal and epithelial, and these cells determine how the tumour grows and spreads. With Metaplastic, the good news is that if it spreads, it doesn't usually spread to the lymph nodes. However, because of the way that a Metaplastic tumour grows, it can spread outwards and have poorly defined edges (so it looks a bit ragged in appearance) rather than a more rounded tumour that most Triple Negative tumours present as. This means that a lot of ladies with Metaplastic breast cancer don't even realise they have a breast cancer until it has grown quite large. Because of its appearance, on scans and ultrasounds it can also look like a fatty mass rather than a cancer, and it's usually only diagnosed with a biopsy. As many ladies have a sizeable Metaplastic tumour when diagnosed, it is typical for a mastectomy to be recommended. This is for two reasons (1) the tumour may be large and (2) in some cases, it will be resistant to some, if not all, chemotherapies. One brighter spot for Metaplastic is that some tumours do show an increase in EGFR (*HER1*) expression, which does provide for specifically targeted chemical interventions. There is a good chance that women fighting Metaplastic breast cancer might benefit from treatment with protein kinase inhibitors. These are definitely things to discuss with your oncologist, who may be able to undertake further investigations. So, generally speaking, the survival rate is no different from other breast cancers of a similar stage.

- **Medullary** – the outlook for somebody with medullary breast cancer is normally very good. Under a microscope the cells will look bigger than other types of cancer cells and will contain white blood cells (something other breast cancer cells don't). Treatment is the same as for a normal type of breast cancer of its main type.

- **Papillary** – Again, it's another rare type that's only found in 1 in 100 breast cancers. This can be found in the duct or be invasive or both, but it can also be benign (non-cancerous). Papillary breast cancers are usually small and compared to more common types of breast cancers and are less likely to involve the lymph nodes. Also, they are more responsive to treatment, and may have a better prognosis than more common types of invasive ductal cancer. It's normally found in older women.

The above are the more usual "rare" special types for Triple Negative but for completeness, I am listing below other special types:

- **Malignant phyllodes** – typically affects older women but is less likely to spread to the nodes and can be cancerous or benign.

- **Paget's disease** of the breast – unlike other types that can be found anywhere in the breast, this affects the nipple and can often be mistaken for eczema, although eczema typically affects the areola rather than the nipple. Essentially this is DCIS of the nipple and is more common in women than men with breast cancer. Normally this is an early-stage breast cancer and is often found in the ducts within the breast but not outside the ducts. It's usually a low grade, slow growing cancer. The outlook is good.

- **Tubular** – although this is only found in about 2% of all breast cancers, the outlook is generally positive as it's normally slow-growing and doesn't tend to spread. It's called tubular because, under the microscope, the cells look like tubes.

- **Cribriform** – this can be "pure", i.e., simply Cribriform or it can be mixed with other types of breast cancer. It can be invasive or ductal but is normally a very low grade (so slow growing), and the outlook is positive with this type of breast cancer.

- **Mucinous** (also known as colloid) – the outlook for Mucinous breast cancer is normally good as this is slow-growing and doesn't tend to spread. It can also affect older women more.

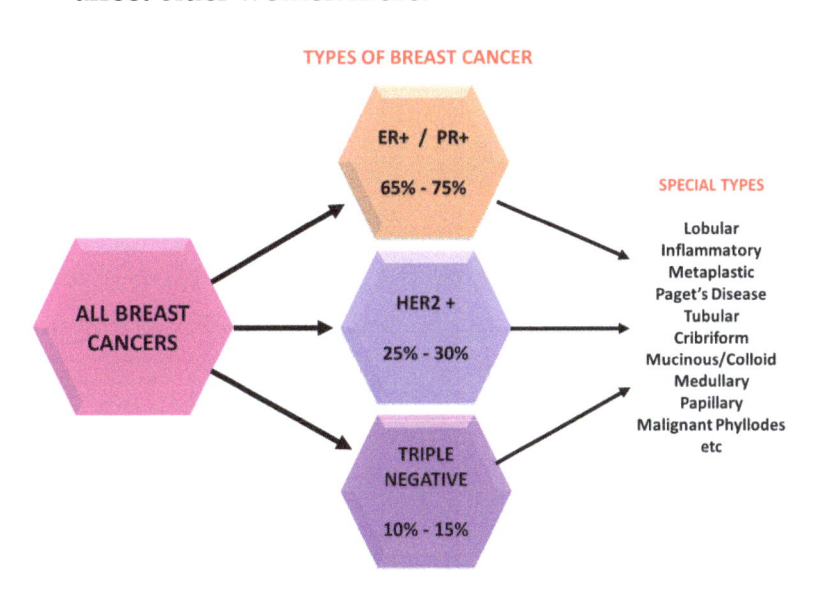

TYPES OF BREAST CANCER

ALL BREAST CANCERS

ER+ / PR+
65% - 75%

HER2 +
25% - 30%

TRIPLE NEGATIVE
10% - 15%

SPECIAL TYPES

Lobular
Inflammatory
Metaplastic
Paget's Disease
Tubular
Cribriform
Mucinous/Colloid
Medullary
Papillary
Malignant Phyllodes
etc

Very Technical – Sub Types of Triple Negative

Just to recap, so far, we've looked at "types" of breast cancer, (ER+, PR+, HER2+ and Triple Negative), and we've also looked at "special types" (the different cellular makeup). So, we know that a Triple Negative tumour can look different under a microscope, but let's walk back a bit. Why does a Triple Negative tumour start – what feeds it if it doesn't have hormone receptors?

This is where it gets complicated because Triple Negative isn't just Triple Negative! It's classed as a "heterogeneous disease", which in layman's terms means a disease that has several root causes and can be "fed" by different things.

I'm afraid this is where science is unavoidable. In 2011, in one of the most quoted research papers on Triple Negative, Lehmann et al. studied Triple Negative tumours and reported that there were 7 different sub-types.

Let's describe this in an easier way. Imagine Triple Negative is a collective term for all sorts of hats – so let's call Triple Negative "headgear". The 7 different sub-types might be (1) a bowler hat, (2) a beanie, (3) a trilby, (4) a cowboy hat, (5) a beret (6) a baseball cap and, (7) something that may or may not be considered headgear, a scarf – 6 are definite types of headgear, all different in appearance, but the scarf is less clear cut and could be used for something else.

Lehman et al, classified these sub-types of Triple Negative Breast Cancer into six different molecular compositions (and the seventh – our scarf - that they couldn't put into a category) as follows:

1. Basal - BL1
2. Basal-Like - BL2
3. Immunomodulatory - IM
4. Mesenchymal - M
5. Mesenchymal Stem Cell - MSL
6. Luminal Androgen Receptor – LAR
7. Unspecified or Unstable - UNS

Almost 70% of Triple Negative Breast Cancers will fall into either the basal or basal-like sub-type.

Why is it important to investigate these sub-types? Well, they all work differently in the body, which means they may respond better to certain types of treatment than others. Typically, most respond to certain chemotherapies called anthracyclines and taxanes (which make up the majority of chemotherapies given as a first treatment at primary diagnosis for Triple Negative). However, if a tumour is not responding as it should, it could be that it falls into one of the less common sub-types, and this may help an oncologist determine your next line of treatment.

Most basal and basal-like tumours have a very high growth rate, but the sub-type, MSL, has low claudin, and this is associated with a slower growth rate. It may be that if your tumour is a grade 1 or 2, it could fall into this sub-type. In the first column of the graph below entitled "characteristics" you'll see that each sub-type has its own set of characteristics, and this helps understand how the cancer grows.

In the right-hand column, it shows the molecular target – in other words which bit of the cell is most likely to be the one feeding the cancer. This is useful because treatments can be aimed at them to turn them off – in a similar way to using

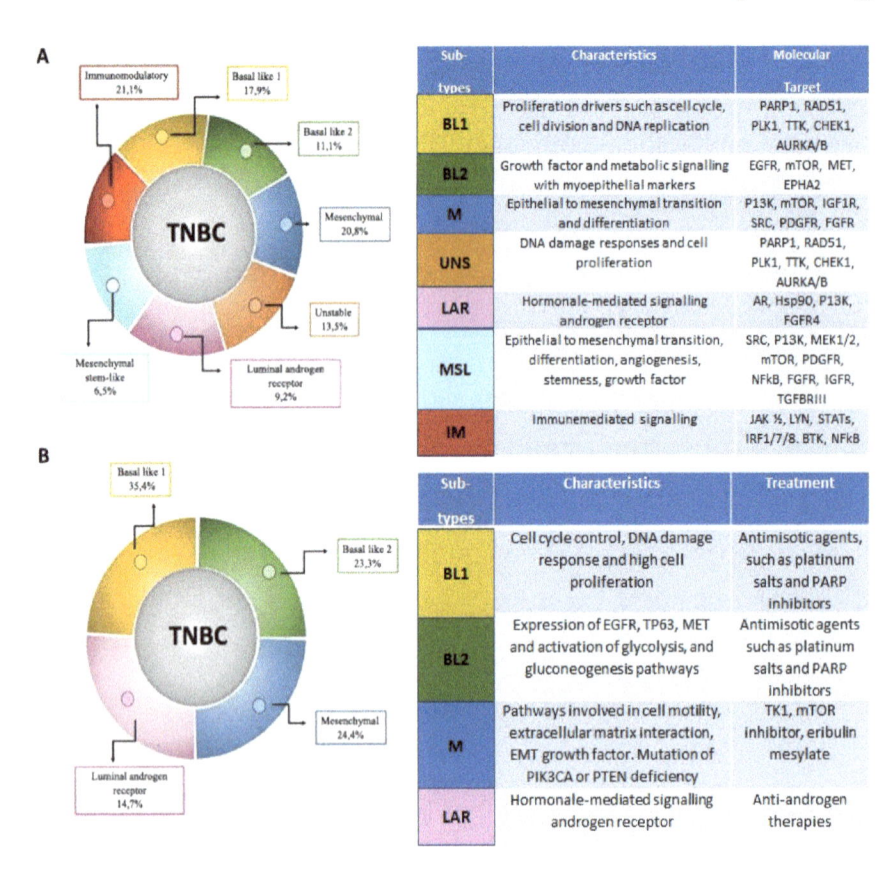

A

TNBC subtypes:
- Immunomodulatory 21,1%
- Basal like 1 17,9%
- Basal like 2 11,1%
- Mesenchymal 20,8%
- Unstable 13,5%
- Luminal androgen receptor 9,2%
- Mesenchymal stem-like 6,5%

Sub-types	Characteristics	Molecular Target
BL1	Proliferation drivers such as cell cycle, cell division and DNA replication	PARP1, RAD51, PLK1, TTK, CHEK1, AURKA/B
BL2	Growth factor and metabolic signalling with myoepithelial markers	EGFR, mTOR, MET, EPHA2
M	Epithelial to mesenchymal transition and differentiation	PI3K, mTOR, IGF1R, SRC, PDGFR, FGFR
UNS	DNA damage responses and cell proliferation	PARP1, RAD51, PLK1, TTK, CHEK1, AURKA/B
LAR	Hormonale-mediated signalling androgen receptor	AR, Hsp90, PI3K, FGFR4
MSL	Epithelial to mesenchymal transition, differentiation, angiogenesis, stemness, growth factor	SRC, PI3K, MEK1/2, mTOR, PDGFR, NFkB, FGFR, IGFR, TGFBRIII
IM	Immunemediated signalling	JAK ½, LYN, STATs, IRF1/7/8. BTK, NFkB

B

TNBC subtypes:
- Basal like 1 35,4%
- Basal like 2 23,3%
- Mesenchymal 24,4%
- Luminal androgen receptor 14,7%

Sub-types	Characteristics	Treatment
BL1	Cell cycle control, DNA damage response and high cell proliferation	Antimisotic agents, such as platinum salts and PARP inhibitors
BL2	Expression of EGFR, TP63, MET and activation of glycolysis, and gluconeogenesis pathways	Antimisotic agents such as platinum salts and PARP inhibitors
M	Pathways involved in cell motility, extracellular matrix interaction, EMT growth factor. Mutation of PIK3CA or PTEN deficiency	TK1, mTOR inhibitor, eribulin mesylate
LAR	Hormonale-mediated signalling androgen receptor	Anti-androgen therapies

targeted drugs for hormonal breast cancers. Unfortunately, this is easier said than done, but it's an area that is researched all the time and is leading to newer advances in treatment options. In 2015, Lehman et al, revised the 6/7 classifications to 4 and the lower graph indicates the changes. It also outlines possible treatment options for each sub-type in the right-hand column.

Using similar classification, the table below, combines treatment therapy from a number of different studies. Some of these are not yet licenced for use in the UK, but it indicates the way forward for future research and potential treatment options.

TNBC TYPE	CHARACTERISTICS	TREATMENT OPTIONS
Basal-like 1 (BL-1)	DNA damage response pathway	PARP inhibitors Platinum compounds
Basal-like 2 (BL-2)	Growth factor signalling, glycolysis and gluconeogenesis	Growth signalling inhibition
Luminal Androgen Receptor (LAR)	High expression of genes related to hormone	AR antagonists
Mesenchymal (M)	Cell differentiation pathway, interaction Between extracellular receptor, mobility of cell	Wnt/β-catenin inhibitors P13K/mTOR inhibitors TGF-β receptor kinase inhibitors
Mesenchymal Stem Like (MSL)	Similar to M sub-type but is claudin-low and high expression of mesenchymal stem cells	
Immunomodulatory (IM)	Immune cell process	Immune checkpoint inhibitors

The above was published in an article on 12th January 2021 by Medicina and the full article can be viewed at https://www.mdpi.com/1648-9144/57/1/62

To recap, and using a similar diagram to ones we've used before, the sub-types of Triple Negative are:

TYPES OF BREAST CANCER

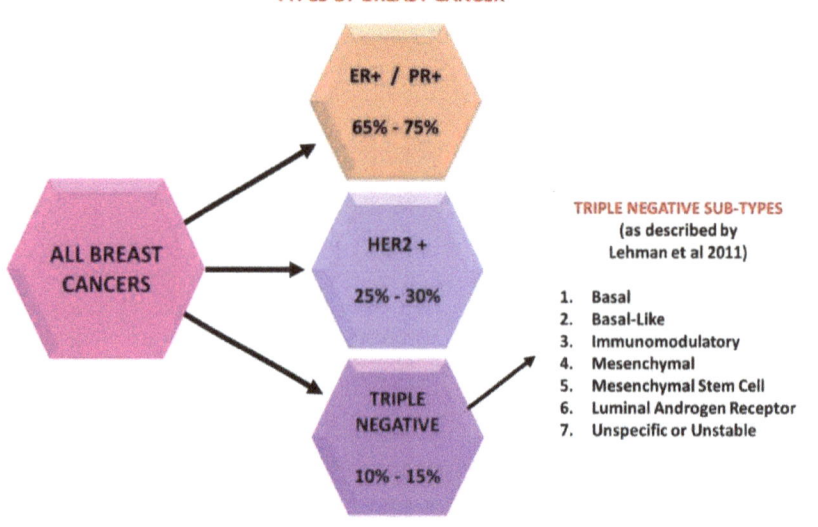

ALL BREAST CANCERS
- ER+ / PR+ — 65% - 75%
- HER2 + — 25% - 30%
- TRIPLE NEGATIVE — 10% - 15%

TRIPLE NEGATIVE SUB-TYPES
(as described by Lehman et al 2011)

1. Basal
2. Basal-Like
3. Immunomodulatory
4. Mesenchymal
5. Mesenchymal Stem Cell
6. Luminal Androgen Receptor
7. Unspecific or Unstable

CHAPTER 8

EMOTIONS

Up until this point, we've explored why and how breast cancer can start, the differences in where it can be found in the breast, and how Triple Negative is different to other types of breast cancer. But what none of that does, is explain how we feel when we're diagnosed – the emotional aspect of a cancer diagnosis.

Feelings at Diagnosis

It's difficult to know how to start this chapter and where to put it in the book. In all honestly, it could feature at any point, but because emotions are heightened typically at diagnosis, and before treatment starts, it seems logical to put this chapter here.

Emotions – both for the diagnosed and that of friends and family – are impossible to predict. You don't really know how you will react, how your friends will be, or how strong your relationships are, until a cancer diagnosis comes into your life. It's an unknown, and definitely not predictable.

When I was diagnosed (and you can read about how I felt in the first chapter in this book), I was floored. Cancer was something that happened to other people. It never occurred to me that I would ever be diagnosed with it. So, my insights into cancer were brief, and I was certainly incredibly naïve as to how cancer could affect me.

When you hear the words "you've got cancer", in my experience, you typically react one of two ways. Either you fall apart immediately, and it hits you like a ton of bricks, or you take it on board and appear to carry on as normal(ish), sometimes falling apart later, sometimes not. There's no right or wrong way to react. Our genes dictate how we respond, and we all have our own protection mechanism.

Our first instinct may be to Google breast cancer or even Triple Negative. This is like walking onto a field, surrounded by snipers all wanting to shoot bullets containing bad news. If you believe everything you read, you'd be convinced you were a walking death sentence, and emotionally this may impact you greatly. The truth is a million miles away, but you need to know where to look, and of course with no prior breast cancer knowledge, starting that journey is a tough one.

I joined a Facebook group for Triple Negative Breast Cancer and on my first day in the group, somebody posted that a lady had lost her life. You can imagine what that did to me! It confirmed everything I'd read on the internet. I cried for days. This was a real-life story, and the lady had died! It took me about two weeks to go back into the group, but it was the best thing I could have done. (A link to the group can be found in Chapter 30.)

I wanted to ask a question and didn't have anybody to ask, so I took the plunge and divided back in! The group were so kind, offering me answers that really did help. In hindsight, I know that posts like the first one I saw are (thankfully), few and far between.

I know there are good and bad groups, but if you find one where the ladies are welcoming and happy to answer any questions you have, and you get comfort from the group, then stay in them. In my experience, ladies in the same position often have the right answers! Don't forget, you will see the occasional bad news post and that must be expected.

Good news, long term survivor posts, are far less common, but this is for a very good reason. After treatment finishes, many will want to forget about cancer, they move away from groups, so there are normally far more "newbies" than long-termers. Thankfully, some long-termers will stay in groups to encourage others.

Let's get back to our emotions and when you were told you had Triple Negative Breast Cancer. For ladies that fall apart, this can include a feeling of disbelief, seeing others happy and getting on with their lives, when you feel you can't. Sleep may be an impossibility, the fear of chemotherapy terrifying, and that's just the tip of the iceberg. How do you tell your friends and family? DO you tell your friends and family? What should you tell them? Should you make a Will? Plan your funeral? And for those with children, just looking at them can be painful, being scared you won't see them grow up, finish school, get married and have babies. Your whole life, and things you wanted to do, suddenly feels impossible and you're in this horrible void that you don't want to be in.

I can't stress enough that unless you've been diagnosed with cancer, I don't think it's possible for anybody to truly understand the horror, and how your world literally changes in a heartbeat. One minute, you're thinking about shopping, going to work, where you'll go on holiday next etc, and the next, you've got cancer and everything else fades into the background and seems trivial and unimportant. Suddenly you're acutely aware of anything cancer related, and you can't get away from it. For example, cancer charity adverts on the television that you probably weren't affected by before, may now become very real. Programmes that raise funds for cancer charities sometimes have real life stories and I used to see them, and they hit home – hard.

Holding in your feelings and grief – because that's what you're going through – can be unhealthy. Life is stressful enough, and cancer on top, can be a catalyst to feeling very vulnerable and alone, so if you need to cry, cry. Allowing the emotions to be felt, and letting them out, can make you feel terrible in the short term, but it can be a release also. For some reason, I used to cry in the shower! I have no idea why because I love taking showers – maybe it was because it relaxed me. I don't know!

There are certain points in the cancer timeline where negative emotions will be at their highest, and the first time is usually the period between diagnosis and the start of treatment, which is a horrible waiting game. You're still processing that you have cancer and then terrified about what's to come, being thrown into the unknown. Once treatment starts, and you have one chemotherapy under your belt, things do get a little easier because you've faced the unknown, and you know what to expect. This isn't the case for everybody, but it's remarkable how many people feel calmer after their first chemotherapy cycle, having experienced the side effects, and knowing what's in store for cycle 2.

Another period when it's common for emotions to be heightened is after finishing the first set of chemotherapy treatments and waiting for the second different set. Again, it's fear of the unknown chemotherapy, and you will settle down again once the new chemotherapy in the second set is over. Before a scan, during a scan, and waiting for results, can also be an exceptionally anxious time, and whilst I can't help you to stop that from happening, I will say that worrying doesn't change the result whatever it may be.

You may not think you're strong but it's remarkable how breast cancer patients dig deep to get through the treatments (and they are testing). There may be very, very, low days where you just want to get off the cancer wheel, and will even consider stopping treatments, but this is where strength is needed. Everybody needs to wallow in grief for a few days, and allow those self-indulgent feelings, but don't allow negative feelings to take over for too long as it's harder to climb back out.

For some, the time after treatment ends is the worst emotionally as you struggle to come to terms with your "new normal" and put cancer behind you. You'll notice that there's a section dedicated to post-treatment in this book. It's nearly always overlooked, and how you feel can come as a real shock. Many people will tell you it's behind you and look forward – but that's far easier said than done. So please make sure you read that section because, hopefully, it will provide reassurance that how you may feel is normal.

Friends and Family

How friends and family react is also important. I have learnt that hearing the phrase "stay positive" was likely to make me scream. That's a phrase I HATE with a passion. For me, having cancer was not something to be positive about. I prefer the use of words such as "strong" or "resilient".

It's not only your own feelings you have to deal with, but it's also how friends and family react. I found that they fell into certain categories – although I'm sure you may be able to add to this list:

1. **Ignorers:** There are people that will ignore the fact you have cancer, or worse still, won't look you in the eye! This makes you feel you have something catching and is absolutely awful. Actually, this is usually because they don't know what to say, and/or, don't want to hear about cancer. It's a very selfish reaction with no thought for you, but they may have their reasons such as having cancer in the family etc. When this happened to me, I decided it was easier for me to avoid them, but that may not be easy for you to do.

2. **Heroes:** These are people that suddenly step up. They bring you food, offer to take you to

appointments or just a shoulder to lean on. They will be the ones that surprise you and give you faith in human nature. It may even be a neighbour who you've never spoken to before, but they see you struggling, and step in to help.

3. **Revellers:** Then there are the so-called friends and family that you can do without and thankfully there aren't many of these! Unfortunately, they want to revel in your misfortune. Maybe they want to be seen as a good friend, helping you, but they don't really care, and they just like having a very ill friend who in turn brings them attention. These are typically people who lead very shallow lives and are jealous of you! Don't be frightened to cut them out of your life. They're not friends if they're like this.

4. **Competitors:** One of the things that always made me laugh was when people told me how ill they were – i.e., having a cold or a muscle strain and there I was, in a wig with no eyebrows, no eyelashes and feeling the effect of chemotherapy! Sometimes you just have to laugh at the stupidity of people! My illness is bigger than your illness!!!!!

5. **Magicians:** Then there's the friend or acquaintance that tells you that cancer has been cured, but the big pharmaceutical companies don't want us to know that. So, they offer a magical solution such as if you take lemon baths or eat less sugar, take dog

worming tablets or a certain pill [insert here any stupid idea that you've been told] you will be cured of cancer! I've often wondered if they would do these things if diagnosed with cancer! I suspect not!

6. **Fatalists:** And let's not forget how some people will tell you about how they know somebody who has died from the exact same cancer as yours! What on earth makes people think this is a good idea is beyond me! Why? Just why? If anything, tell the cancer patient a good uplifting story or just don't say anything! I don't want to hear about Auntie Mabel who suffered from horrible breast cancer for years and then died a painful death! I'm not Auntie Mabel and neither are you!

When you look at the above, you'll wonder who the sane person is! Well, it's you! However, all these things can take a toll on your mental health. You will probably focus on the negatives, and that's part and parcel of this journey I'm afraid. Don't let this get you down. Take time to re-evaluate things, where possible surround yourself with the people who are in your life for the right reason and ignore those who aren't.

What about your family? Well, there's a saying that you can't choose your family, and unfortunately, not only can they fall into the 6 categories above, but whereas you can walk away from friends, it's a bit more challenging if they're part of your family.

Having cancer can be a strain on our loved ones. They can feel powerless and don't know what to say or do, and this can make them seem uncaring and thoughtless. Sometimes they shut down and don't want to talk, which can be difficult for you. Or at the other end of the scale, they become over-protective to the point where you're not allowed to do anything – which can be just as frustrating if you want to at least try to do some things!

Unfortunately, it can cause marriages to end as it can put an unbearable strain on an otherwise sound marriage. Sometimes, it's the catalyst for a marriage to end and for some, the ending of a partnership can come out of the blue and make a stressful time even more difficult. It's an unexpected side effect of this horrible thing called cancer, but for some, they will come out stronger and find happiness in other areas and even perhaps with a new partner.

I'm fortunate to have an amazing husband, but even he was sometimes a bit naive about what I needed. When I was diagnosed, I told him I didn't want to be treated like a cancer patient. I wanted everything to be as normal as possible. He took me at my word and so didn't help with the cooking (which he used to help with before), the washing, the cleaning, taking our daughter to school etc., and by the end of my second chemotherapy, I was on my knees with exhaustion! I burst into tears and yelled at him that he obviously didn't care about me because he wasn't helping at all! He looked at me horrified and said, "But you told me you didn't want to be treated any differently to normal" and yes,

I did, and he was doing exactly that! We then had another chat, and not only did he help, but in all honesty, he did the lion's share of the chores. So, my point here is that you do need to talk. Our families are not mind-readers. If you need help, speak up. Hopefully there will be people that will be there for you.

Other than my family, my "one person" was ironically the one person I didn't want to tell about my cancer! My best friend Nicki is like a sister to me. Our lives have run in parallel for years and about 12 months before I was diagnosed, Nicki's mum was diagnosed with breast cancer (HER2+). Nicki was devastated by her mum's cancer, and I just couldn't face telling her that the same thing was happening to me. One day, I slipped up when speaking with her. I can't even remember how the conversation went, but she suddenly stopped mid-sentence and said to me "What do you mean?", and I realised I had to tell her. She was SO angry that I hadn't confided in her, and I think if the roles had been reversed, I'd have felt the same, but it seemed like the right thing to do at the time.

From the day Nicki found out, she was there for me. She lives at the other end of the UK but would just turn up on my doorstep! She made sure her visits coincided with my chemotherapy appointments so she could give my husband a break, she made me laugh to the point where I couldn't laugh any more by taking the mickey out of my headgear (don't worry that sounds mean but it's not – it's the way we are together). She likened my look, when I was wearing my beanie, to Wee Willy Winkie! And most of all, she was there when I had my low points. She didn't judge. She just listened and then made sure that for the next few days she'd check up on me. Everybody deserves a Nicki in their lives, and I hope your Nicki gives you as much comfort as mine did.

Telling people you have cancer can be difficult, and you may not get it right but, the one thing I would urge you not to do, is to tell your friends and family in a group. This can associate getting together as a group, in the future, with bad news, and might worry people unnecessarily. Also, it may stop people from asking questions – especially children. It's far better to tell people one on one wherever possible and change how you tell them to suit the person. This is, of course, exhausting for you, but it does encourage people to ask you questions further down the line.

If you have children, how they react to your diagnosis can be a big concern and they can really have a tough time – and I'm not just talking about young children. Older children too. Depending on their age, they may understand what's going on or they may not. For the older children, dealing with their emotions can be very challenging. They may never have thought of the possibility of losing you and suddenly they are confronted by it. Your GP can recommend some great services who will help with counselling or group therapy, and it may be something you want to suggest (at the appropriate time).

For younger children, there are a few books that are available to help parents explain, in very simple words, what's happening to Mummy and some schools have very good teachers or a school nurse that can help.

A good book, aimed at younger children, called "Mummy's Lump" helps to explain to children in a non-frightening way, what's happening and why. Hair loss can be one of the issues that a child struggles with and Barbie have made a doll that hasn't got hair, and this may be something you might want to use. In addition to the Barbie doll, a charity called Cancer Hair Care (details can be found in chapter 30) offers free hair loss dollies to help children understand hair loss during cancer treatment. Each knitted dolly has hair on one side and can be turned upside down to become hair free – there are also cute little hats and scarves for the children to play with. The dolls are adorable and if you have young children, this is a lovely way to introduce them to what may happen.

Another idea is to get a few pebbles and together with the child, decorate them. The parent keeps the one that the child has decorated and vice versa. The idea is that the parent is always with the child via the pebble, and when the child is stressed or anxious, they can hold the stone or cuddle it. There are so many ideas to help, but these are just a few.

However, it may not be plain sailing. Unfortunately, some children, can rebel or react in a way you wouldn't expect AND at a time when you really don't need it. My own daughter, who was 12 at the time, was fine for a few months but as she saw me going through treatment, it was as if a switch was flipped, and she became rebellious and did everything she could to be badly behaved – not consciously, of course. I vividly remember going to her school parents' evening and walking from teacher to teacher being told how awful my, previously well-behaved, daughter was. It got to the stage that the last teacher said to me "I wish I could tell you something positive about Katya, but I can't". Can you imagine, you're going through cancer treatment (which all her teachers knew by the way), feeling dreadful from chemotherapy, worrying about dying and trying to pretend to the world that you're fine and hearing that? It was all a bit too much, and if there was a very low point for me, it was that.

Needless to say, I spoke to our GP, and we agreed that my daughter needed some counselling because it had got to the stage that she wouldn't even say the word cancer. She would walk out of the room if anything cancer-related was being discussed, and she literally closed down. She had counselling with Macmillan but unfortunately wouldn't open up (I don't think she really liked the counsellor), but it was a safe place that she could talk if she wanted. Thankfully after a year of being the child from hell, she completely turned around, and I can honestly say, I'm now the proudest mum of the best daughter in the world! They say that time is a healer, and it certainly was in our case.

In fact, one of the happiest days of my life and one I'll never forget, is when she turned eighteen and asked "Mum, what day did they tell you, you had beaten cancer?", and I had to tell her that there wasn't really a day because I hadn't been told that. So, she asked, "what date was your last treatment – the day I got you back". I asked her why she wanted to know, and she said she wanted a tattoo with that date on it, a tiny one, so she could have it with her forever. I'm not a fan of tattoos, but for her to even speak about cancer in the way she did, made me realise that she had most definitely come out the other end, and it really touched me.

I've mentioned counselling above and I think it's really important to say that counselling can be a lifeline for a cancer patient at any point (even during treatment). However, ESPECIALLY after treatment it may be needed, and I'd encourage you, to read the chapter on what happens after treatment. Accepting you have cancer and then moving on can be incredibly difficult. I had counselling with Macmillan, and I don't know if I was just lucky but my counsellor, Cat, just "got me". She really helped me to understand how I was feeling and what I could do to move forward, which I was finding incredibly difficult. Please ask for help if you need it. It may or may not work for you but it's somebody neutral to talk with.

Another way of helping to deal with emotions can be to take anti-depressants. I was really surprised that it's incredibly common for cancer patients to be given these. Again, I would urge you to visit your GP or reach out to your cancer team if you're struggling to cope. There's absolutely no shame in it. Cancer can be a problem too big to bear and you might need a bit of help to take the edge off.

There are also meditation and calming apps that may help, especially if you're having trouble sleeping. Also, perhaps do some yoga if that's what you fancy.

Body Image

Whilst this may not be an issue straight away, a negative body issue can definitely occur. When we have breast cancer, there's nearly always a surgery involved. This will give us scars that can be a powerful, and a constant reminder of what's happened. There's no getting away from it. We may also have surgery that will change the way we look. Our breasts are integral to us being female and for some ladies, this change can overwhelmingly affect how they feel about their bodies. They may feel unfeminine, unattractive, different, and are living with "killer boobs".

For some, they may be very definite in what they want from surgery, and it can be really difficult if a patient has different expectations from what is being offered by the surgeon. This can be very upsetting. If you feel strongly that you are not being listened to, or not getting what you need, asking for a second opinion can be useful. It will allow you to either find a viewpoint that is a closer match to your own, or will give you clarity on what you can, and cannot, be offered. NHS care is excellent but often surgeons are working to pre-set rules which can be relatively restrictive – and the same restrictions apply in the private sector.

Having a lumpectomy usually can't be avoided with breast cancer but having a mastectomy, for some ladies, is very difficult to come to terms with. As part of the mastectomy process, I had to see a psychotherapist, and she asked me to tell her exactly why I wanted a mastectomy, what reconstruction I wanted and why. I explained all my reasons, told her about the downsides there might be, and how I'd researched what could go wrong. She was satisfied that I had looked at all options, carried out the research, and understood the risks and benefits, but I was very sure and confident in my decision.

Interestingly, she told me that the ladies she saw who were unhappy with their outcome, were generally the ones who hadn't really looked into the chosen option, or who hadn't had a say in what they were having because they were told by their surgeon what they would have. In some cases, a mastectomy is unavoidable. Some ladies were also shocked at the size of their breast after reconstruction and found it difficult to live with smaller or larger breasts than they had before. There are so many variables, and until you're faced with them, it's impossible to know how you'll feel.

For a positive body image moving forward, it's key that the decision-making process should be a partnership between you and your surgeon. You need to understand each other's viewpoints and find a solution that works for you, and your surgeon is happy to provide.

When Things Go Wrong or Not to Plan

Delays in Treatments

Unfortunately, with such a long treatment timeline, things can take unexpected turns. Most patients will experience a change to their initial plan, but this can have a knock-on to how you feel. Delays are very common, but can be totally unexpected, and you may feel that you're not coping, especially if it happens more than once. For ladies struggling with anxiety already, when treatment gets delayed, it can send minds into overdrive. There's a common fear that a few weeks delay in treatment will mean the cancer will spread. It won't. It's highly unlikely to make any difference to your overall outcome. The only time that delays may be problematic is if a delay is 12 weeks or more, however, your oncologist will probably have a solution for you.

Scans

If you're experiencing aches and pains, or have an unexplained symptom, your oncologist may order a scan just to be cautious. Having scans is a stress-inducing part of the process especially if they throw up something. Oncologists don't like to scan us too often, because having them, really does bring on "scanxiety". We worry before we have the scan, during the scan and then the wait for results is never quick enough, and it feels like we're being diagnosed all over again! Scans can also throw up things that are totally normal for us, but not for the next person. Also, scans show up every little nodule or node that may be inflamed – this can be because we've had our flu injection a few days before, or have had our covid vaccination, or we may just be under the weather, and our nodes are inflamed whilst they're fighting off the infection! However, once these show on a scan, they need more investigations to screen out cancer. Many ladies have nodes in their lungs they were blissfully unaware of and it's just a normal finding. I can't tell you how many ladies have this! The only way to know for sure is that if they don't respond to chemotherapy, they are usually not cancer and are just part of us!

I had a scan once that showed a "ripple" in my abdomen – lots of investigations later, it was concluded that nothing was wrong at all. The CT scanner had just had a blip as it was filming me! However, the stress this caused was enormous!

Not being heard or listened to

Having a good team you trust is really important. If you feel you're not getting on with your team, you can ask to switch (if there's another team available at your hospital). If you don't want to do that, you may need to change hospitals if there's another near you. If the level of care you're receiving is really upsetting and you feel that you're not being looked after, you can make a formal complaint. Each hospital has a Patient Advisory Liaison Service (PALS), and they can always step in and help. Thankfully, the majority of hospitals provide a good level of care. Before you decide to change your team, make a list of why you're unhappy with the care and ask to speak to your oncologist or surgeon. Often, just getting things out in the open can be helpful.

I would also urge you to check with other breast cancer patients whether your care is "normal" but don't compare line by line. We are all different, and there will be differences in treatment plans, frequency of scans etc. However, basic care should be relatively the same. Sometimes our expectations are too high, and it could be that our care is normal, but our expectations aren't.

CHAPTER 9

PREPARING FOR CHEMOTHERAPY & SURGERY

Things to Do Quickly

This chapter is intended to be suggestions only, and for the time period when you're waiting for treatment to start. You may want to invest in one or more of the suggested items or even none! Everything listed below I found helpful, but I'm sure everybody has a different list of items they would add!

Eyebrows

This is not for everybody but when you lose all hair during chemotherapy, there is nothing that will stop you from losing your eyebrows. Only a very small proportion of ladies keep their brows. Eyebrows and lashes are typically the last hair to go, and it can be weeks into your treatment before you look in the mirror and realise your brows (and lashes) have gone missing!

Eyebrows frame your face and without them, if you try to draw them on (for example) it's quite easy to place them too high (so you'll look surprised), too low (so you look angry), or just draw them on too much (and end up looking like Coco the clown)! If you feel that you may need a little help in this area, and want to look a bit more like your old self, you can have your eyebrows microbladed BEFORE treatment starts.

Microblading is a semi-permanent type of make-up that uses a form of tattooing so that when your hair disappears, you're left with tattooed eyebrows. That sounds incredibly scary and probably conjures up very false looking eyebrows in your mind, but they can look very natural as the beautician will probably use hair strokes, so there isn't a block of colour. There are several different methods for applying the ink to your skin, but you will normally have an anaesthetic cream applied to your brow area to numb them first. It will still be a little painful, but it's bearable and doesn't take very long. The colour will fade over time (it's individual, so I can't be more precise), but typically, they will last until your natural brows grow again. You can't have microblading, or semi-permanent make-up, done during chemotherapy because this can be dangerous by causing an infection, but before chemotherapy it's fine.

Lots of beauticians will offer you a reduced rate and, in some cases, even treat you for free if they know why you're having it done. They will normally follow your natural brow line so that when your hair falls out, you will be left with eyebrows in the right place. With microblading, you normally have a top-up after a few weeks, but you may not be able to have that, depending on your timescales. Don't worry, you can have this done after treatment ends if you want (you may not need it). Please make sure that you only go to a recommended beautician though.

I had my eyebrows microbladed before chemotherapy, and it was the best thing for me. They did fade slightly but thankfully looked natural, and it was one less thing to worry about.

Teeth

Please visit your dentist before treatment starts. You need to make sure that any work is carried out before chemotherapy starts. This is essential. I've included a section purely on teeth, so please read that to find out why it's essential.

Thermometer

You will be asked, all through treatment, to keep an eye on your temperature. A high temperature can be an indication of an infection or neutropenia (explained in the chemotherapy chapter), and it's essential you keep an eye on this. Moreover, if you want to take painkillers (they will mask a temperature), you will be told to check your temperature beforehand. There's no need to buy a fancy thermometer, but if you can afford it, it's worth buying two – only because one may go wrong or need batteries, etc., so having a backup is a good idea.

Visit Your GP

If you have a friendly GP, it's worth visiting them for a few reasons:

There are certain side effects that you may get during treatment and having medications in the house to treat them can stop you from worrying and panic buying, when treatment starts. The items I would include are diarrhoea and constipation remedies, lubricating eye drops (Hyloforte is a good one), a mouth wash with an anaesthetic (Difflam was the one I found helped most, but Biotin is another good one), either Duraphat toothpaste or Biotin Toothpaste.

If you're in England, you are eligible for free prescriptions when diagnosed with cancer (Scotland/Wales/Northern Ireland have free prescriptions). Your GP can give you a form to fill out (your oncologist/team may also give you this). Fill this in and send it off. It gives you free prescriptions for five years, but it DOES NOT cover dental charges, unfortunately.

Free Chemotherapy Kit

Cancer Support UK, and a few other charities, offer a free "chemo kit" for those newly diagnosed. The kits comprise a range of products, including toothpaste, hand gel, notebook and pen, alcohol-free mouthwash etc. Details can be found on their website, and their address is listed in Chapter 30.

Pillows For After Surgery

After breast surgery (all types), you may be advised to sleep in a sitting position. This can be really difficult, propped up by a million pillows behind you. I found the large V-shaped pillows (you can find them on Amazon and elsewhere) much more comfortable, and I used two behind me. I then used normal pillows down each side to stop me from turning on my side. You may not need the larger pillows, but the suggestion is there if you need it! I also used mine during the day when I was watching television, to give a bit of extra support. There is also a charity providing free heart shaped pillows to use after a mastectomy. They're called Pillow Pals, and a link to their Facebook page can be found in chapter 30. These are really cute, and I've seen ladies take them to their chemotherapy sessions too.

Bedding/Pillow Covers

Whilst I'm talking about sleep, during chemotherapy you will be plunged into menopause so cooler cotton bedclothes (or even those made from bamboo) may be a little more comfortable. If you don't want to buy those, the one item I would suggest is a silk pillowcase (they are surprisingly cheap on Amazon). If you're cold capping, a silk pillowcase will be kinder on your hair, and it will also help to keep the head and neck cool.

Bras to Wear After Surgery

Whether you have a lumpectomy or mastectomy, if you're having surgery you may want to shop for post-surgery bras. If surgery is before chemotherapy, it's worth looking for these quite quickly. As a breast cancer patient, the VAT will be removed from the normal price and online shops will deduct this at checkout. You may have to fill in a form to confirm you're a breast cancer patient.

You normally wear a supportive, sports-type bra (no underwires) after surgery 24/7 for 4-6 weeks (depending on what your surgeon tells you). My advice is that because these bras must be worn at night, for comfort, you may want to opt for a back size, one size larger than you are now. You also may experience some swelling after surgery, so if it's too tight, it can be uncomfortable.

There are so many different types on the market, and it can be hit and miss as to what suits you. My favourite "daytime" bra was from Marks and Spencer, and I wear it to this day (clearly new ones bought over the years), and the night-time option was a button front, unattractive but very supportive bra. Make sure you try all the bras on because in my experience they don't always follow normal sizes as accurately as they could, and you need to make sure they're comfortable A front fastening bra (for ease of getting on and off) is recommended, but if you find one that's a back fastener and comfy, you can always fasten it at the front and then gently spin it around to the back.

Hair

Please see the chapter on hair, cold capping etc. This section is purely a shopping list! If you are cold capping, you may want to invest in a kind shampoo and conditioner and wide-tooth comb. Waterman's shampoo and conditioner are specifically developed for hair loss, and I had remarkable results with the shampoo (although I wasn't as keen on the conditioner). They also have an elixir that you can use on your scalp. Also, Olaplex shampoos and conditioners are used by lots who are cold capping, so this may be worth investigating.

For those who are not cold capping, other products recommended by patients are Lush shampoos and bars, and shampoos from the Body Shop that are mostly natural. Biotin and Plantur33 are products that you should only use after treatment ends as they contain chemicals and can be detrimental during chemotherapy. It may also be worth having a look in your local health food shops for ideas.

Supplements

Do NOT take any supplements, without speaking to your team beforehand. There are certain vitamins and minerals that can cause issues during treatment. Your team will approve anything you're already taking but anything new, please run past your team.

Headwear – Turbans, Scarves, Wigs, Hats etc.

You may want to invest in headwear (especially if it's winter). Looking for these before treatment, does allow you to practice (especially with scarves and turbans). There's more information in the chapter about hair.

Nails

Please see the section on nail care in this book for information, but you may want to invest in a very dark (as close to black, or even black) as possible nail polish OR some cuticle oil.

CHAPTER 10

QUESTIONS TO ASK YOUR ONCOLOGIST/SURGEON

Your First Meeting

So, we are now at the point where treatment will be starting but what will it be like? At your first meeting with your oncologist or surgeon you may want to ask questions but it's difficult to know what questions to ask! If you are allowed to take somebody with you, please do because it can be confusing, and you may not remember everything. You could also buy a notebook and take it with you to all appointments (and use it before each appointment to write down questions as you think of them). Some oncologists will allow you to record the meeting on your phone, but some don't, but of course, you need to ask their permission.

Use as many or as few of the following questions you think may be helpful. Both lists assume you're seeing the consultant for the first time – if you've had surgery first, some of the questions you may already know by the time you see your oncologist and vice versa:

Questions for your Oncologist:

- What size is the tumour, and is there evidence of node involvement?

- What's the stage of the cancer?

- What's the grade of the tumour?

- Does the biopsy show anything unusual for example a specific type of Triple Negative?

- Will I be tested for defective genes such as BRCA1 and 2?

- For younger ladies who may want children in the future - please use this opportunity to ask what options may be available. You may want to ask about the effects on fertility and whether Zoladex would be appropriate. (This is a long-acting hormone that is used to put a woman into menopause for a short time. This is called ovarian suppression. You could also ask about freezing embryos or eggs).

- If you are interested in taking part in a trial, ask if there are any relevant open trials.

- What will the treatment plan be i.e., type of chemotherapy?

- How many cycles of chemotherapy will that be and how often? (Sometimes it's weekly, fortnightly, three weekly or a combination).

- When are blood tests carried out prior to each cycle? (This is usually the day before or on the day of chemotherapy, but it's a good idea to check so you can plan, especially if you work or will need childcare etc).

- Are there facilities to cold cap? (If you want to)

- Does the hospital offer the possibility of using cold gloves and slippers? (Not many hospitals do)

- How often will you review my case/see me?

- Will there be scans and, if so, when?

- If you are on any tablets, check that your oncologist will allow you to take them - so go with a list of your medication/supplements.

- If you are diabetic OR have any pre-existing medical conditions that might mean you shouldn't take steroids, please mention this.

- If you are post-menopausal (not chemotherapy-induced), ask if you will be given Bisphosphonates (see chapter further in the book)

- If you are pregnant/breastfeeding, you may want to ask about what precautions or differences there will be to your treatment and why.

These next questions may be answered by your oncologist OR breast care nurse:

- Who should you contact if you are feeling unwell? Typically, there's a "chemo hotline" but each hospital has its own procedure.

- If you haven't already got the form to complete for free prescriptions – (England only – not applicable for Scotland, Wales, and Northern Ireland where prescriptions are free) ask if they can give you one.

- Are you given a voucher for a wig? If yes, do they have contacts with a local wig shop etc?

Questions for your Surgeon:

- What's the size of the tumour, and is there evidence of node involvement?

- What's the stage of the cancer?

- What's the grade of the tumour?

- Does the biopsy show anything unusual for example a specific type of Triple Negative?

- Will you be advising a lumpectomy or mastectomy and why?

- If given a choice, ask, in your case, what the difference would be.

- If you have a larger tumour that's going to be removed by lumpectomy (before chemotherapy), will you be able to have anything to plump out the breast and avoid a dent?

- Will you need full node removal (in some cases you may need to)?

- In the case of mastectomy, you may want to ask the following questions:

- o Is it possible to have an immediate reconstruction?
- o What type of reconstruction does your surgeon offer? Surgeons usually specialise and you may need to see other surgeons if you want a specific type of reconstruction. If your surgeon doesn't offer the type of reconstruction you're interested in, ask if he/she would be able to refer you to somebody else for a consultation.
- o If having a reconstruction, is it possible to keep the nipple and have a free nipple graft? Only some surgeons do this – if your cancer is near the nipple, it's not a good idea.
- o Are there options for nipple tattooing/nipple mounds?
- How long is my recovery likely to be?
- When will I be able to drive?
- Do you use breast drains after surgery and if yes, how long do they stay in for?

When am I classed as cancer free?

This is a question that lots of ladies want to know and it's worth asking your oncologist and surgeon but don't be surprised if you get different answers! Years ago, we were told "you're in remission" however, this terminology is no longer used. The preferred wording now is "no evidence of disease" and sometimes you'll be told you are cancer free.

But at what point does that happen? We know with Triple Negative, we want to get to the five-year stage when our chances of a recurrence are greatly reduced, but when does that timeframe start?

Interestingly, there isn't an agreed timeline! The options are:

- The date of diagnosis – this makes no sense to me because you still have cancer in your body so how can your cancer-free timeline start at this point? However, some oncologists will suggest this is the correct date.

- The date all treatment ends – again, this makes no sense because some ladies will have surgery/chemotherapy (in any order) then radiotherapy and sometimes more oral chemotherapy. This means that treatment can last for a very long time but some of it is purely a belt and braces approach because the cancer is no longer in the body. Whilst I understand how this may be a date you'd want to use, potentially, the clock won't start ticking for quite some time even though you may have no evidence of disease in your body.

- The date of surgery – this is the date I use, and it's because at this point, we know that the cancer tumour (and any affected nodes) is out of the body.

You are therefore technically cancer free. Any treatment you have after surgery is a mop up for cells that may, or may not be, in your body.

It's up to you what date you use, and there are no right or wrong answers so either go with what your team suggest or use one of the above if you feel more comfortable with it.

Copy Letters / Reports

There is a new national policy that patients should be provided with copy letters. If you do not want to be copied in, please mention this to your breast care nurse – some people prefer not to see facts in black and white. However, if you're not being copied in, please speak with your nurse, who will be able to help.

CHAPTER 11

SURGERY OR CHEMOTHERAPY FIRST?

As mentioned in an earlier chapter, after your diagnosis has been confirmed, you'll be assigned both an oncologist and, also, a surgeon. What you'll find is that we are all (quite rightly), treated as individuals, and so it's at this point that our care may be different from the next person. You may have surgery first and then chemotherapy, OR you may have chemotherapy first and then surgery. The decision will be made by your team when looking at your diagnosis. As a very rough benchmark, the majority of teams will apply the following criteria to decide your treatment plan, but I must stress, there may be reasons why this differs, and it could simply be your consultant's choice!

It's important to also stress that it doesn't matter which order you have treatment, as it all does the same job. There are pros and cons to each.

Surgery before Chemotherapy (Adjuvant)

As a general rule, if you have a small tumour (under 2cm) with no or limited node involvement, you might be offered surgery first. The term for having surgery before chemotherapy treatment is Adjuvant.

The advantage of surgery first is that the cancer is out of your body and has no chance to do any more damage. Chemotherapy is then a "mop up" to catch any cells that can't be seen on scans. The downside is that because the tumour is out of your body, there's no way to tell if chemotherapy would have worked on it.

Chemotherapy before Surgery (Neo-Adjuvant)

Normally, chemotherapy before surgery is given where you have a larger tumour and definite node involvement, and this is referred to as Neo-Adjuvant. The disadvantage to this option is that if you have chemotherapy first, you're leaving the cancer in your body for longer, which potentially means it might spread if the chemotherapy isn't working, BUT this option gives you the power of knowing if chemotherapy is working, which is an advantage. If chemotherapy isn't working, your oncologist may decide to move you to a different type of chemotherapy, or even move to surgery and then back to chemotherapy.

If your nodes are affected, then it's a good idea to know that chemotherapy has done its job.

The other advantage is that if you have a large tumour, it would be difficult to perform a lumpectomy at surgery as, removing a large tumour may take away too much of your breast, that would be challenging to rebuild. So, to try to get you to the stage where a lumpectomy may be possible, chemotherapy is given first to shrink the tumour. If it does the job, then it might eliminate the need for a mastectomy which, for many ladies, is a distinct advantage.

CHAPTER 12

SHOULD YOU HAVE CHEMOTHERAPY?

Yes – absolutely 100% you should. There are exceptions, for example, if you have an existing medical condition, that means having chemotherapy would be a significant danger to your overall health, BUT if that doesn't apply, my personal opinion is that chemotherapy saves our lives, and without it, we're playing Russian Roulette. Many ladies have pre-existing conditions but still have chemotherapy. So having a disease or illness normally doesn't rule out treatment.

There is a worrying trend in America that ladies (who have any type of breast cancer) that's 10mm or less, will only be offered surgery and radiation. What I find inconceivable is that Triple Negative is not differentiated from hormonal breast cancers. We already know that Triple Negative is typically more aggressive and has a higher recurrence rate, AND we can't take tablets after treatment has ended to prevent a recurrence. So, for me, this decision is absolutely unacceptable, but in America, a lot of treatment is driven by cost – thankfully, in the UK, this is less of a concern.

There is also a trend that is creeping into the UK of oncologists giving a choice to patients of whether they have chemotherapy or not. Now let's look at this logically – imagine you've just been diagnosed, the only knowledge of chemotherapy you have is what you see on the television and let's face it, that doesn't paint a pretty picture and can be frightening. You're sitting in front of the oncologist, your head is in bits, you're trying to find out how to survive, and you're given the choice of having chemotherapy or not!!!!!!

To me, this is not something that should happen. A newly diagnosed patient will think, if they're being given the option, it means the cancer isn't too serious, and so may not be necessary. I can absolutely see how that happens, and I'm in a group on Facebook where I see newly diagnosed ladies going through this exact situation. If given the option, please talk to your oncologist and ask them, if they had Triple Negative, what they would do. They're the experts – we're not!

My own personal belief is that anybody with Triple Negative who can have chemotherapy, should absolutely go for it, and let me explain why …………

Chemotherapy Isn't Just for the Tumour

Chemotherapy treats the **WHOLE** body. Radiotherapy and surgery only target a specific area. In earlier chapters, I've mentioned that we can have cells that are unseen on scans because they are just too small. So, what if you've got some escapee cancer cells that are on the march around your body? Radiotherapy and surgery won't get to them, but chemotherapy will. Chemotherapy is our friend, not our enemy, because it can get to those cells and potentially stop them in their tracks!

You may believe that my thinking is overkill but remember, we don't know all the ways that cancer spreads, and even small tumours can throw off rogue cells. Do you want to refuse chemotherapy and risk the chance of cancer coming back? At that point, the choice of having chemotherapy or not may be too late.

What If I Only Have A 3-8% Benefit If I Have Chemotherapy?

When my surgeon wrote to my GP and said I had a 5% chance if I had chemotherapy, I thought, why on earth should I bother then? I thought it meant that I only had a 5% chance of living, even if I had chemotherapy. It doesn't mean that at all! It's a little bit complex, but I hope the following makes it clearer.

Surgeons and oncologists use a tool called Predict (that you have access to as well - https://breast.predict.nhs.uk/tool) where they put in your statistics and out pops what percentage your LIFE SPAN will be increased by if you have chemotherapy or not. It compares your likelihood of surviving breast cancer, to the rest of the population. This is about survival, not having another breast cancer or rates of spread.

My surgeon kept asking me if I wanted to know my predicted survival rate, but I wasn't ready to deal with the numbers if they were anything under 100%! Actually, the highest score in a 5-year period is 98%, so nobody gets 100% so I was never going to achieve that! It's assumed that at least 2% will die from non-related breast cancer issues, but I was too scared to find out my survival rates until I was quite far into my treatment.

However, please bear in mind, at the end of the day, they're only statistics and it took me over a year after diagnosis to visit the website and punch in the numbers. If you're feeling wobbly, don't do this, because it's still frightening to see the numbers no matter what they are. Typically for Triple Negative, the percentages you will be given range from 3% to 8%, and your percentage will be based on your individual circumstances.

If you decide to fill in the tool, and you're not sure what each section means, click the info button next to the question and it'll guide you. The one that you may not know is the Ki67 value. If you're unsure, click the box for "positive", as it's likely to be the correct one.

The Predict tool gives you results for a 5, 10, and 15 year period, and my 5 and 15 year survival results are shown here. Interestingly, I have no idea why, radiotherapy is not included in the final result panel!

Let's look at my results:

Imagine there are 100 ladies. In 5 years, the statistics show that 2 ladies would die from non-related breast cancer issues. So, we now have 98 ladies. If you look at the table, the results gave me a 5% added benefit when having chemotherapy and an extra 2% for bisphosphonates discussed in a later chapter - so it means:

| Table | Curves | Chart | Texts | Icons |

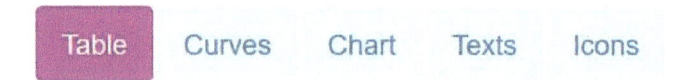

These results are for women who have already had surgery. This table shows the percentage of women who survive at least | 5 | 10 | 15 | years after surgery, based on the information you have provided.

Treatment	Additional Benefit	Overall Survival %
Surgery only	-	84%
+ Hormone therapy	0%	84%
+ Chemotherapy	5%	89%
+ Bisphosphonates	2%	90%

If nobody died from breast cancer, 98% would survive at least 5 years. 🛈

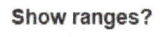

Show ranges? 🛈   Yes   No

- If I had surgery only, my chances of survival in the group of 98 ladies would be 84%.

- I can't have hormone therapy because I had a Triple Negative breast cancer so, that doesn't add anything to my result.

- If I have chemotherapy, I get an added benefit of 5%, which means my survival rate goes up from 84% to 89% out of 98%. So, it's getting better.

- If I have bisphosphonates after treatment, that's another 2%, so my percentage has now gone up to 91% (it's rounded down in the table). So basically, out of 98 women, I have a 91% chance to still be around in 5 years. If I had surgery only, I would have an 84% chance which is quite a bit less.

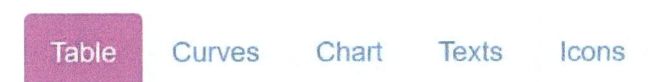

Table   Curves   Chart   Texts   Icons

These results are for women who have already had surgery. This table shows the percentage of women who survive at least 5 10 **15** years after surgery, based on the information you have provided.

Treatment	Additional Benefit	Overall Survival %
Surgery only	-	70%
+ Hormone therapy	0%	70%
+ Chemotherapy	7%	77%
+ Bisphosphonates	2%	79%

If nobody died from breast cancer, 90% would survive at least 15 years.

Show ranges?   Yes   No

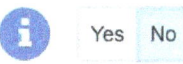

The percentage changes over time as we get older, and people die of natural causes etc - so let's look at the 15 year statistics. In 15 years, it's expected that the death rate will increase because of natural causes, so we now only have 90 ladies.

- With surgery only, out of 90 ladies, my chances of survival would be 70%. That's quite a dip.

- As I can't take hormone therapy, the additional benefit is 0%.

- So, what happens if I have chemotherapy? My survival percentage increases to 77%.

- Another 2% is added on for bisphosphonates so that increases to 79%, so, I'm now only 11% less than somebody who hasn't had breast cancer. That's so much better than 20%!

- This means that out of 100 ladies (the same age as me) in 15 years' time, 10 will die of natural causes but out of the remaining 90 ladies, I have a 79% chance of still being alive, compared to 70% if I didn't have chemotherapy or bisphosphonates. That's only 11% less than somebody who hasn't had cancer.

So bottom line? Chemotherapy will improve your life expectancy more than if you only had surgery.

Will Chemotherapy Prevent Recurrence/ Recurrence Statistics?

It's important to state that the percentage mentioned in the above section, ONLY references the benefit of chemotherapy to your overall survival. It is NOT a measure of the likelihood of a recurrence. There is no tool to predict recurrence rates.

What is the risk you'll have a recurrence and what does recurrence mean? Let's start with the second part of that question. A recurrence is when your current breast cancer comes back after treatment has ended, likely caused because the cancer cells haven't been completely eradicated first time around. A biopsy, examined by a laboratory, will be able to tell by the make-up of the new tumour if it is a recurrence, as opposed to a brand-new breast cancer.

A new tumour, if not a recurrence, is a totally unconnected breast cancer. This would be called a new primary breast cancer as opposed to a recurrence. Some ladies will have breast cancer, once, twice, or even three times and a mixture of recurrences or new primaries. Don't forget, so long as it's contained in the breast and/or nodes, it's treatable and curable.

For the purposes of this section, I will use the word recurrence to describe a recurrence, and a new primary.

What are our risks of recurrence? Unfortunately, that's a complete unknown. Without chemotherapy, the risk is likely to be higher. There may be other risk factors such as how well (or not) you've responded to chemotherapy, the sub-type of Triple Negative you have etc – but these are all unknowns with respect to recurrence rates. Frustratingly, there have been no large breast cancer studies looking at recurrence rates for many years. And there has been nothing specifically for Triple Negative.

So where does that leave us? We need to look at scholarly articles and small(er) scale trials and investigations. Annoyingly, if you look online, there are many articles focussing on Triple Negative, and the results vary from stating a recurrence rate of 7% right up to 50%! They all use different parameters to gauge their percentage, which means there's no level playing field either. That's not helpful, is it?

So, what's the truth? In my experience, some oncologists in the UK will quote a recurrence figure of around 25% (which would include a recurrence, new primary or spread of the original tumour to other organs). This is probably about right if you take the average of all the scholarly studies. To see if I could quantify the percentage, in 2019, I set up a poll in the Triple Negative Facebook group and from those that responded, about 25% had had a recurrence/new primary/spread. Of course, this is a smaller sample of Triple Negative ladies, but it does bear out the average recurrence rate might be around 25%.

Before you start panicking – please bear in mind that the statistics mean 75% will NEVER have another brush with breast cancer. It will be a thing of the past for the majority, and don't forget, these are just statistics!

CHAPTER 13

CHEMOTHERAPY

In this chapter, I'm going to discuss chemotherapy, the different regimes and what to expect. The chemotherapy outlined below is typically used for primary breast cancer, i.e., when it's first discovered in the breast and/or node area only. If you have breast cancer for a second time, or it spreads later, different chemotherapies will be used, but I'm going to concentrate on the chemotherapy regimens that are used at the moment, for a primary diagnosis.

It's very, very, important to note that chemotherapy regimens vary from hospital to hospital, and even from oncologist to oncologist. Although there are NICE guidelines in England that suggest the minimum and types of drugs to use, it's up to the oncologist as to what you'll be given. The recommended minimum has been proved to deal with cancer, and you will certainly get that, but anything over and above is a bonus.

So, what exactly IS chemotherapy? Simply put, it's a way of killing cancer cells using chemicals. The use of chemotherapy to treat cancer began at the start of the 20th century when it was discovered that a side effect of a drug that had been used during World War 2 for its chemical properties had the ability to kill cancer cells. It wasn't until the 1960s that it became clear that the use of chemotherapy, when added to surgery and radiotherapy, could cure patients with various advanced cancers. From there, chemotherapy has steadily become the drug of choice for many cancers, including breast cancer.

Chemotherapy has become synonymous with cytotoxic chemotherapy (i.e., toxic, or deadly to cells) used for cancer treatment, but its original use was to treat Tuberculosis. As many drug treatments for cancer are not all cytotoxic chemotherapy (in the old-fashioned sense), oncologists tend to use the term systemic anti-cancer therapy now (SACT). This may be a term you will see used, but for the purposes of this book, I will refer to treatment as chemotherapy.

Which chemotherapy will work varies from one person to the next. Think of it like this – if you broke your leg, would the break be in exactly the same position and at the same angle as for somebody else? The answer is probably not. However, you will both have broken legs, and the treatment is usually the same but may need some tweaks here and there.

With Triple-Negative Breast Cancer, it's the same, because our tumours can be different, as mentioned in an earlier chapter. Some tumours will respond to one chemotherapy better than another, but the majority will react to at least one in a cocktail of drugs. This is why we don't just have one chemotherapy drug; it can be 3, 4, 5 or even 6!

Due to its toxicity, most chemotherapies have a lifetime limit that a patient can receive – or at least a suggested amount that shouldn't be exceeded. This is because if you have too much, it can end up causing other problems on top of cancer. However, there are always solutions and there are lots of different drugs that can be used so don't panic and worry you'll run out of options.

Typical Chemotherapy Regimes

There are various regimes for early breast cancers, and they can be used together or apart. Detailed below are the more common regimes, but please bear in mind you don't have to have them all! Also, the order in which you have them doesn't matter – chemotherapy is chemotherapy, no matter when it's given.

Chemotherapy is divided into different "types"; anthracyclines, taxanes, platinum-based and anti-metabolites. Typically, patients will either respond better to anthracyclines or taxanes. It's impossible to tell in advance. So, the purpose of giving a combination of drugs is to ensure the patient gets the best possible coverage.

The dose of each chemotherapy is tailor-made for you and will be based on your height and weight. This is why, at most hospitals, you are measured and weighed before each session. Don't compare your dose with anybody else because it's unlikely to be the same!

Using your height and weight as a measure for the drug dosage doesn't mean you'll be able to cope with 100% of the recommended amount. Sometimes, the dose is intolerable, and you may need it adjusted. If you are finding that side effects are too bad, then each drug can be reduced, and this will be anywhere between 75 and 100%.

However, I have seen lots of ladies say they can't cope with the side effects, and they're going to ask for a reduction. I need to stress that for some, chemotherapy can be very tough (other ladies have an easier time of it), but unless you REALLY can't bear it, I would urge caution in having a dose reduction. It's a short-term pain and will be a distant memory at some point. Ultimately, your oncologist will make the decision.

Turning back to chemotherapy, in no particular order, the acronyms of the drugs used are as follows, and you'll find a description of each following the list:

Anthracyclines:	FEC or EC or AC
Taxanes:	Paclitaxel or Docetaxel
Platinum-based Antineoplastic:	Carboplatin
Anti-metabolite:	Capecitabine (also known as Cape or Xeloda). Capecitabine is not given to everybody and there's a section on its use below.

FEC/EC/AC (Anthracycline) Chemotherapy

Each letter stands for a drug that makes up a set of chemotherapies given together – so, for example, FEC is a combination of 3 drugs; EC only uses 2, as does AC. The drug names are:

- **F**luorouracil
- **E**pirubicin
- **C**yclophosphamide
- **A**driamycin (also known as Doxorubicin hydrochloride)

Interestingly, many oncologists are now dropping Fluorouracil from the FEC set of drugs as a large study, conducted in 2015, concluded that adding the "F" drug into the combination wasn't actually giving many benefits and, in fact, might result in a higher incidence of side effects. Therefore, it is more common now that EC is given. The "E" drug, Epirubicin, is often called "the red devil" because it's red and discolours your urine for the first few hours after you've had it, which can be worrying unless you are aware of the side effects.

AC uses the same C drug (Cyclophosphamide) as both FEC and EC but replaces the F and E drugs with Adriamycin. Interestingly, AC was once the preferred treatment, but as FEC and EC became more popular, it was replaced. However, there has been a resurgence in the use of AC, and it is just as good as the other combinations.

FEC, EC or AC are normally given once every 3 weeks (called a cycle), with all drugs given on the same day, but in a few hospitals, it may be given weekly and even fortnightly.

The dose will be the same over the whole period, but it will be adjusted so that you get more or less in any one infusion.

Each cycle, you will have these drugs, one after the other, in an infusion via a cannula, portacath, or PICC line (see below). Typically, you will have either 3x3 weekly cycles or 4x3 weekly cycles. So, a likely maximum time frame is either 9 or 12 weeks from start to finish with this set of chemotherapy drugs (assuming no delays).

Docetaxel, Paclitaxel, Abraxane & Carboplatin Chemotherapies

For the other set of drugs, you will normally have a drug that belongs to the Taxane range of chemotherapies either with or without a platinum-based chemotherapy, as follows:

- Docetaxol
- Paclitaxel
- Abraxane (also known as Nab-Paclitaxel which may be used in exceptional circumstances to replace Paclitaxel)
- Carboplatin (platinum-based and optional)

You will either be given Docetaxel OR Paclitaxel OR Abraxane. The main difference is that usually Docetaxel is typically given once every three weeks, Paclitaxel and Abraxane are given weekly. However, Docetaxel is now sometimes given on a weekly or fortnightly basis.

There is a risk with a taxane (specifically Paclitaxel) that you will have an allergic reaction which is why you are normally given an antihistamine before your chemotherapy session begins (via an infusion rather than a tablet). For your first few chemotherapy sessions, a nurse may administer the dose manually or will sit with you to make sure you don't have an allergic reaction. It bears mentioning, to reassure you, that allergic reactions are quite rare, but if they happen, your infusion will be stopped and, depending on your reaction, restarted in a different way.

There are a few ways of administering the chemotherapy after you've had a reaction, and that's to slow the rate of the infusion, which seems to work for many ladies. However, if it doesn't, then the drugs will be stopped, and Paclitaxel may be replaced by Abraxane. Abraxane is Paclitaxel that has been manufactured in a slightly different way and is coated to protect you from an allergic reaction. This drug is incredibly expensive – I was once told it's £10,000 per infusion, and whether that's correct or not, I don't know – but I do know that it is ONLY given to those who have a definite allergy.

In addition to a taxane, you may be given Carboplatin. It has become more common to see this in a regime, and the change has happened since 2019. Not all hospitals use it though. When it was first introduced into the breast cancer setting, it was thought that it worked better for ladies who had a genetic mutation such as BRCA1 and 2. Further trials demonstrated that it could also work for ladies without a genetic feature, so it has crept into the standard care at many hospitals.

Carboplatin is generally given on a three-weekly basis. So, if you have Paclitaxel weekly, every 3rd week, Carboplatin will be added in. As with the other drugs in the first section, you will either have these drugs for a maximum of 9 or 12 weeks, depending on your oncologist.

Typical timescales for chemotherapy

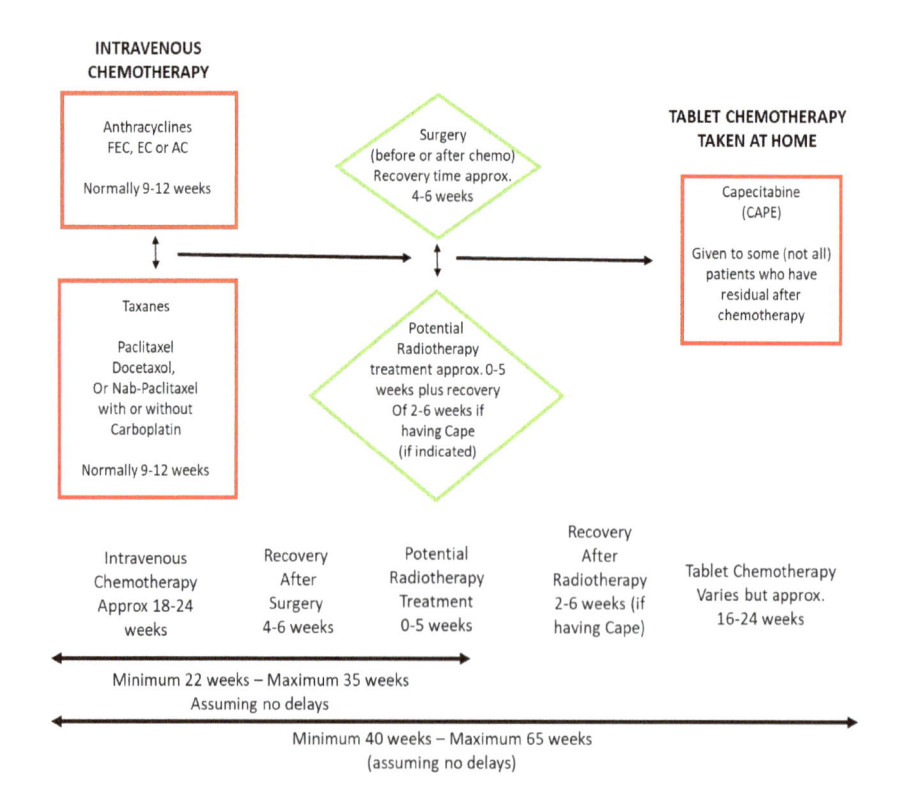

INTRAVENOUS CHEMOTHERAPY

Anthracyclines
FEC, EC or AC

Normally 9-12 weeks

Surgery
(before or after chemo)
Recovery time approx.
4-6 weeks

TABLET CHEMOTHERAPY TAKEN AT HOME

Capecitabine (CAPE)

Given to some (not all) patients who have residual after chemotherapy

Taxanes

Paclitaxel
Docetaxol,
Or Nab-Paclitaxel
with or without
Carboplatin

Normally 9-12 weeks

Potential Radiotherapy treatment approx. 0-5 weeks plus recovery Of 2-6 weeks if having Cape (if indicated)

Intravenous Chemotherapy Approx 18-24 weeks

Recovery After Surgery 4-6 weeks

Potential Radiotherapy Treatment 0-5 weeks

Recovery After Radiotherapy 2-6 weeks (if having Cape)

Tablet Chemotherapy Varies but approx. 16-24 weeks

Minimum 22 weeks – Maximum 35 weeks
Assuming no delays

Minimum 40 weeks – Maximum 65 weeks
(assuming no delays)

If you look at the timescales, it indicates that your chemotherapy will not be any longer than 24 weeks. HOWEVER, this does not account for any stoppages or delays because of infections, illnesses etc., etc. Nearly everybody going through chemotherapy has a "blip" where treatment is delayed for one reason or another. For example, I developed a life-threatening infection just after my 4th EC. Before starting the weekly Paclitaxel, my oncologist told me I had to have a break of at least four weeks to recover and get my strength back. It was a good idea because I did feel stronger when I got back on the hospital wheel again, but what it did mean was that my overall treatment lasted longer, and the goalposts kept moving, which was difficult. I need to emphasize, and I've said this at various points in the book – do not allow delays to worry you. Chemotherapy carries on working in your body, and to reassure you, I had delays of 8 weeks in total.

What if Chemotherapy Doesn't Work/Only Partly Works?

Unfortunately, as mentioned earlier, chemotherapy is difficult to predict how it will work for you.

It is very common that one set of chemotherapy drugs will work better on your tumour/nodes than the other. So, for example, you may have limited or no response to the anthracycline set of chemotherapy, but your tumour will respond well with the taxane regime. It could also be the other way around! It's impossible to predict.

Ladies sometimes have very high expectations and expect at the end of all chemotherapy that their tumour will have disappeared, and they will be told they have no evidence of disease remaining (NED). In reality, this happens to only a few, and it's far more usual for there to be some tumour shrinkage, or at the very least, the tumour remains the same size. If this happens, it doesn't mean that chemotherapy hasn't worked. On the contrary, it hasn't grown, so the chemotherapy has stopped it in its tracks and so has partially worked.

Ladies also get hung up on the size of their tumour, thinking that this indicates the response to chemo, especially if they know the starting measurements and then have a scan at the midway point. It can be an indicator, but it must be borne in mind that most scans are not 3D, and they only provide a guide to size. Also, some tumours, as they die, don't shrink. They can even grow, even though they're inactive. This is called pseudo progression. Other reasons why a tumour may not shrink are that although the active cancer cells have been killed off, what remains is a scar or necrotic (dead) tissue.

So, what you want to see is no tumour progression and possibly some shrinkage. Clearly, anything better than that is excellent!

If you don't have complete shrinkage, the tumour/nodes may or may not have active cancer cells remaining, and this is where the next step in chemotherapy comes in, and Capecitabine may be given.

Capecitabine (Xeloda)

If I had been writing this book five years ago, Capecitabine ("Cape") wouldn't have been mentioned! It is now part of the normal regime at some hospitals, but ONLY for some patients, not all. As mentioned above, Capecitabine is an oral chemotherapy that may be given after chemotherapy, surgery, and radiotherapy (sometimes before radiotherapy) IF there is residual cancer that has active cells in either the tumour and/or nodes.

Why is it not given to everybody? Well, there are two reasons. The first is that there is still limited long term data to its effectiveness and secondly, if there's no cancer after chemotherapy and surgery, what would the Capecitabine work on? It's assumed all cancer is out and stray cells have been dealt with. Having Capecitabine is introducing another level of toxicity to your body which would be overkill if it's not going to help. If you don't have Capecitabine this time round, it's in your back pocket if it might be needed at a later date (hopefully not).

Unlike the other chemotherapies mentioned above, Capecitabine is in a tablet form to take at home, but before it's given to you, you will have a couple of tests to determine how it will suit you. One of these is a blood test to check for an enzyme called dihydropyrimidine dehydrogenase (also known as DPD). If you have low levels of DPD, it may indicate that you are likely to suffer from severe side effects from this drug, and your starting dose will be lower than someone with higher levels. Very low DPD levels may mean the risk to your health in taking Capecitabine outweighs the benefits, so you may not be given it.

Like the other chemotherapies, you will take the tablets in cycles, possibly with a week off and, just like intravenous chemotherapy, will also need blood tests prior to each cycle to ensure that you are coping with the drug. The number of tablets and cycles you have will be determined by your oncologist, and again, it will be individual for you.

There are two side effects that are most common with Capecitabine, and they are tiredness and a condition called hand/foot syndrome. Whilst there's not much that can be done about tiredness other than to reduce the dose, hand/foot syndrome can be controlled. The symptoms are really painful hands and feet that may be red, sometimes swollen, very sensitive, and the skin may peel off (although that won't necessarily be painful). The way to stop this is to ensure you lubricate your hands and feet every day with a good moisturiser. Double Base Gel is exceptionally good, but others recommend Udder Cream. There are also other moisturisers that your GP can prescribe, and if hand/foot syndrome does develop, they should be able to give you a cream to help settle the symptoms.

The good news with Capecitabine is that you are unlikely to lose your hair, which is always a positive.

So, we've looked at the various regimes but what's the actual process of having chemotherapy?

Before Your First Chemotherapy Session:

You will probably have your blood and blood pressure taken, as well as height and weight, as these give a starting baseline for you and what's "normal". In addition, you may have an ECG and liver/kidney function tests (usually just with a blood test). Sometimes a bone scan may be ordered. The tests are individual and will be based on what your oncologist thinks you need, and these are one-off tests.

In addition to the initial tests, before each chemotherapy session, you will have your blood taken and you may be weighed – either the day before or on the day of chemotherapy. The reason for doing this is to make sure before each cycle that you're well enough for treatment.

How is Chemotherapy Given to a Patient?

Your first type of chemotherapy will almost certainly be a liquid so you will be hooked up via a needle in your arm called a cannula or via a Portacath or Picc line (see below) for the infusion.

Before the chemotherapy is administered, you will probably have a saline drip to clear the vein and ensure the line is working properly. This only takes about 5 minutes or so, and also, antihistamines (again an infusion rather than a tablet) may be given 15-30 minutes before the chemotherapy. Depending on the chemotherapy drug you have, you may be given an injection in your tummy called Neulasta/Pegfilgrastim/Filgrastim to help with neutrophils –

please see the section on G-CSF injections for more information and an explanation as to why they are needed. Steroids and anti-sickness tablets are also given, but when you take them and in what form depends on the drugs you're being given.

So, back to chemotherapy .... many ladies have chemotherapy by IV infusion using a cannula in their hand/arm. However, chemotherapy is an irritant and sometimes this can cause damage to the veins. If this happens, your team may suggest the use of a central line instead of a cannula, and these are called Portacaths and PICCs, but what are they, and why might you want/need one?

A Portacath or PICC is a way of avoiding veins by inserting a tube into your arm or chest and administering the chemotherapy through that. That sounds very scary but it's not! Different hospitals have preferred lines, so it's difficult to predict which you may be offered. These lines are short-term and left in for the duration of your treatment, but they can also stay in for years after too!

Differences Between PICC and Portacaths

The main difference between the two is that a Portacath is totally under the skin, usually positioned on your chest or (less frequently), on your arm. The PICC sits above the skin and is usually sited somewhere on your arm. Of course, there are pros and cons for each, but the main advantage of having a Portacath is that you can hide it, go swimming and, as it's under the skin, there's less chance of infection. Because the PICC sits above the skin, it's more prone to infection and does need to be protected when showering etc. However, a Portacath will cause a scar (approximately 1-2" long) where it's put in and taken out, but the scar with a PICC is considerably smaller.

Portacath (Power Port / Port)

As mentioned, the Portacath sits under the skin but, in most cases, does create a small lump. Under the skin sits a triangular-shaped device with a soft centre. In order to inject the chemotherapy, a needle is pushed through your skin and enters the soft centre of the port. This is almost painless, with just a slight pushing sensation. The chemotherapy is then injected and flows from the port via a tube that takes the chemotherapy up towards the neck and down towards the heart, where it circulates around the body.

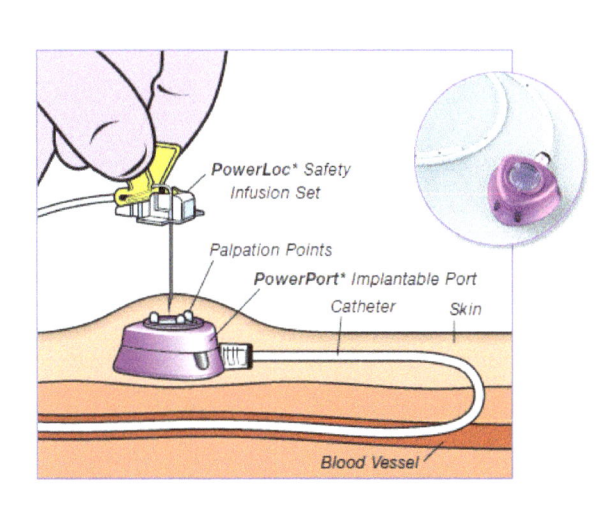

Prior to having a PICC or Port fitted, you may be asked to wash with a specialised skin wash that removes bugs! Don't be offended if you're asked to do this – it's to eliminate the risk of infection. The wash doesn't smell too bad, and you need to wash your hair with it also.

To insert a Port, you will meet a specialist radiographer who will assess you for a suitable place to insert it. It must be an area that has sufficient coverage (i.e., fat)! When a site has been agreed, you'll be put into a gown and taken to a theatre where they have a machine that is part x-ray/part scanner but only small. You lie down on the bed, and the radiographer will examine the area and give you a local anaesthetic.

Once you're suitably numb, an incision is made, and the port is placed under your skin. You feel a bit of tugging and pulling but nothing more. For some people, a small incision is also made in the side of the neck to allow for the tube that goes inside from the port up to the neck to be inserted correctly. You may feel a pop as this is done, but again, it doesn't hurt.

When the port is in place, a dye is injected to ensure that everything is working as it should be. If it's all in order, the incision is sewn up, and you can get off the bed and back to the ward. From start to finish, it probably takes 30 minutes, and the thought of it is probably more daunting than the reality.

It's best to allow the port to settle for a few days before using it, but it can be used on the same day if required. Prior to each chemotherapy, your nurse will inject saline to ensure that the port is not blocked before beginning your treatment.

One thing that did happen to me is that because of where my port was, it did twist slightly, and the pipe became kinked. My nurses were really struggling to get blood out or anything in, so I had to pop back to the theatre for about 30 minutes, where the doctor pushed and prodded me and got it to work! There was no cutting involved that time. I think I must be an awkward patient because only one of the nurses could ever use my port, and luckily, she was there throughout my treatment! Most people have complication-free ports!

If you look at the picture of the port, you'll see there are three bumps that guide the nurses where to insert the needle. There are different types of ports; some have these bumps, others don't.

PICC Line

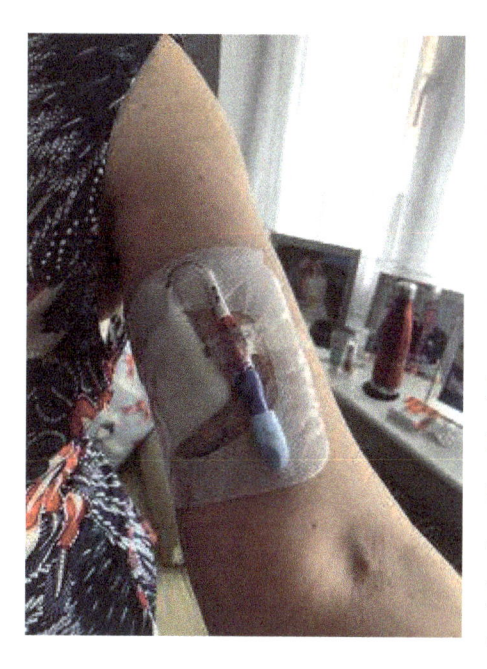

The main difference between the PICC and Portacath as mentioned above, is that with a PICC, the access point is permanently on top of the skin (although it does have a cap on it when not in use to prevent infection). Since there's an element that is open, you have to be careful during washing. If the

PICC line is on your arm, you're usually given a sleeve to put over it for protection.

PICC lines require flushing with saline and also Heparin, to avoid blood clotting, more regularly than the port, but this is carried out by your breast care nurses or a district nurse if needed.

Inserting a PICC line is a bit easier than a port. After numbing the area, a small incision is made in your arm, and a thin tube inserted into a vein which then is gently moved towards larger veins nearer to your heart. This is usually done with the aid of a type of scan to ensure correct placement. Once it's confirmed to be in the right place, dressings, and a cap to the end of the line are put on to keep it in place. A lovely lady, Kim Roberts, has kindly given me permission to use the image of her arm with a PICC line inserted.

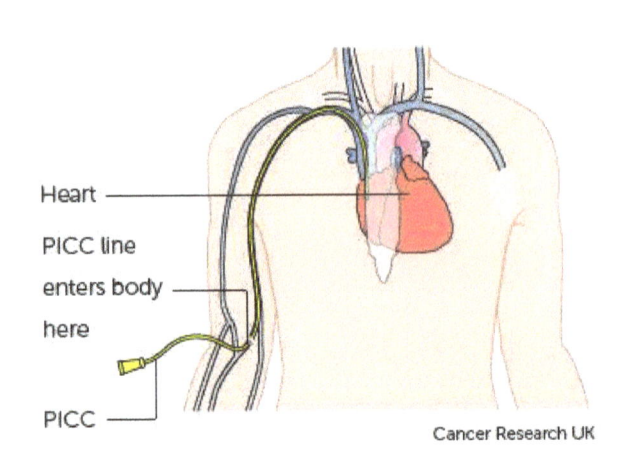

One thing to be aware of is that the dressings covering the PICC can irritate the skin. There are a few options and different ones to try, so don't suffer in silence if your skin becomes sore. Also, occasionally, a PICC line will come out a bit. If this happens, there is a small lock type device that can be added for extra security.

Removing the Lines

Oncology teams like to keep lines in (whichever one you have) until treatment has finished, and they know that it won't be needed anymore. They are designed to be in your body for many years, but I couldn't wait to have mine taken out. The procedure to take it out is very simple and much quicker. For a portacath, you go back to the side theatre, and it's removed, and you're sewn up. Again, there's some prodding and poking but nothing graphic or anything frightening. It's actually pretty straightforward and can be a relief if you hate your line like I did! I used to call my port my alien, and although I loved how easy it made the treatments, I wasn't as keen on having it in my body!

PICC lines are just as easy to remove and can be taken out either in theatre or on the ward by a qualified nurse.

Steroids

To help with side effects, you may be given steroids. The more common steroids are:

- hydrocortisone
- dexamethasone
- methylprednisolone
- prednisolone

Steroids will usually be given on the day of chemotherapy with instructions on when to take them. They are normally in tablet form, although they can be injectable also. Steroids are only taken for a short while during each cycle to help with side effects. The main issue with steroids is that they may cause a red face (which disappears after a few days), and appetite may increase, but the most common side effect is not being able to sleep. This usually happens when a patient takes their steroids from lunchtime onwards. The earlier you take the tablets, the less likely they are to affect your sleep.

If you're taking the tablets before 9am but still struggling to sleep, it might be worth speaking to your team because they can change the steroids to another to see if they suit you better.

If you are diabetic, please speak with your endocrinologist and ask them to liaise with your oncologist. It may be that they will remove steroids from your treatment plan. Steroids can cause your blood sugar levels to be unpredictable and high. I'm a type 1.5 diabetic and reliant on injectable insulin, and my team agreed that I shouldn't have steroids. So, it is possible to get through chemotherapy without them if needed.

Common Chemotherapy Side Effects

As if having cancer isn't bad enough, chemotherapy can be cruel, and there are certain side effects that are unavoidable. That said, for every side effect, there's a tablet or a solution, so if you're suffering, speak to your team. Don't wait until your next appointment.

Although I've listed the most common side effects further in this chapter, it's highly unlikely that you will have them all! You may be lucky and only have one or two, but I've detailed the main side effects for information purposes.

Don't forget that even when you're having treatment, you may still get colds, flu, viruses, covid, muscle strains etc., and sometimes they run alongside and make you feel poorly. A rule of thumb, with all side effects, is that if something is unbearable, call your team RIGHT AWAY. However, if it's a "niggle" like a muscle strain, it is better to wait a week or two and see if it calms down.

Side effects with a three-weekly regime normally start either on the first day or may be delayed for a few days, but the first ten days are when you'll potentially feel at your lowest. Days 11 to 21 are usually a bit easier.

G-CSF Injections – Neutropenia

Unfortunately, especially if you're needle phobic, one of the medications you will need are G-CSF injections. You will be taught how to do them, and injections are usually in your tummy area. If you struggle and really can't do them, a family member can be shown how to do it, and if all else fails, a district nurse may be available to help. These injections are what's called granulocyte colony-stimulating factors, and they are drugs that help prevent infection during chemotherapy. These are really important as they help to increase the number of white cells in your blood (neutrophils).

Chemotherapy can attack bone marrow which means fewer white blood cells are produced, and with fewer white blood cells, your ability to fight off infection is compromised. Injections are normally given for the first few days after chemotherapy and can be anywhere from 1 to 5 days. Bone pain is the most common side effect of these injections but can be relieved with over-the-counter antihistamines and painkillers (although please check your temperature first as you should not take painkillers whilst having chemotherapy unless you are absolutely certain you don't have a temperature). Also, do not take antihistamines without asking your breast care nurse. The typical brands of injections are called Filgrastim and Pegfilgrastim – there are other brands, but these are the two most commonly used.

Unfortunately, for some, these injections help but don't help enough and you may become quite poorly with low neutrophils. It's quite common for low neutrophils stopping a chemotherapy session until you're well enough. However, there is a natural product (a particular brand of honey) that does appear to help with neutrophils for the majority that take it, and I include details in section Chapter 27 if you would like to read more about it.

Damage to Veins

A fairly common side effect with chemotherapy is damage to veins as mentioned above, and this is normally when chemotherapy is given via a cannula. This can be a short or long-term complication. When this happens, the vein or an area where the veins are, may rise to the surface and look brown, or you'll see a raised lump. The way to know for sure is that if you try to straighten your arm, it will feel tight, like it's pulling inside and will be painful.

After my second chemotherapy, with a cannula, a vein in my arm became very painful, and I was told I couldn't have more chemotherapy without a central line. I was offered a Portacath, and although the idea of it was awful, in practice, it was one of the best things I had. Not only could I have chemotherapy via it, but I could also have my blood taken for testing, which meant fewer needles. Thankfully my vein did repair itself, but it took about 6 weeks to get back to normal and I found putting a hot water bottle on the area really helped. If you are having chemotherapy via a cannula, I would urge you to keep an eye on your veins. If you start to see evidence that your veins are suffering, please let your team know as soon as possible. If the vein is continually used, after it's shown signs of damage, it can become a permanent side effect.

Nausea

Nausea is one of the most common side effects, and thankfully there are quite a few drugs to combat this. If one doesn't work, your team can always change you to another. Medication varies from tablets that you only take on the day of chemotherapy, to ones that you take for a week or two (or a combination of both). I was given Akynzeo, which at the time of my treatment, was a relatively new drug. I took one tablet half an hour before chemotherapy and then didn't have to take anything else. I have to say that I only felt a slight level of background nausea throughout my treatment, so it definitely worked for me. Emend is another recommended drug. Please don't suffer from nausea – speak to your team about a change of medication if you're suffering from this.

Peripheral Neuropathy

Peripheral neuropathy typically occurs more with the taxane line of treatment than the anthracyclines, and it is something that breast care teams will keep a close eye on. Peripheral neuropathy is the feeling of tingling or numbness in the hands and feet. If bad, it can creep further up the legs, but this is in quite severe cases. Normally your team will either stop treatment for a short while, to allow you to recover, or will reduce the dose of chemotherapy. If left unchecked, it can be a side effect that takes a long time to reverse and, in some cases, it can't be reversed. This doesn't happen to many people, but it is something to be aware of.

Some hospitals provide cold gloves and slippers that are put into a freezer and changed every 20 minutes. You wear these during your treatment, and it discourages the chemotherapy from getting to your hands and feet, which in turn stops, or lessens, the neuropathy. Because these are time-consuming, bulky and a freezer is required, not all hospitals have the facility to offer this. I believe that cold gloves and slippers can be purchased from Amazon, and I have seen cases where ladies have stored them in their freezer at home and then taken them to treatment in a chiller basket. I'm not sure whether this works or not, but if you're suffering and want to try it, it might be worth giving it a go. If you do get peripheral neuropathy, there are certain drugs you can be prescribed to relieve symptoms, so don't suffer in silence.

Other common side effects

The most common side effects will either occur straight away or may build up over time. This is a list, but it doesn't mean you will have all, or any, of them!

- Hair loss – this was perhaps one of the worst side effects of chemotherapy for me. Not because I'm vain, but because losing my hair meant that I looked like somebody undergoing treatment. Some ladies find it completely liberating, but I wasn't one of them. You can try to keep your hair by cold capping, but it doesn't work for everybody. If it doesn't work for you (and it didn't for me), you are entitled to a free wig, or wig voucher, and if you don't want to wear a wig, there are lots of lovely scarves, turbans, and headwear that you can buy. Please see the chapter on cold-caping and hair for more information.

- Watery Eyes – when eyelashes go, eyes may start to stream uncontrollably, become itchy and cause soreness around the eyes from constant wiping. This is (bizarrely) called Dry Eye Syndrome. It will resolve once the eyelashes come back, but in the meantime, ask your GP to prescribe lubricating eye drops such as HyloForte. Using a warm compress/heat mask, specifically for eyes, also helps. This is a temporary side effect and unlikely to be permanent.

- Tiredness – there's not much that can be done about this, but you do need to rest as much as possible and tiredness is to be expected. This can also build up, the more treatment you have. If you need a nap during the day, please do so, because you need to recharge your batteries.

- Sore mouth/teeth – Please see the chapter on Teeth and Chemotherapy. A mouthwash with a small amount of anaesthetic can help with a sore mouth (Difflam is a good choice). Brushing teeth with a soft toothbrush and allowing the brush to do the work and a specialist toothpaste such as Duraphat or Biotin will also help. You may experience a dry mouth. If you do, Biotene make a mouth lubricant (and I'm sure there are others on the market), that can help with this.

- Headaches – these can feel like a hangover headache and are very common for the first week after chemotherapy. A good over the counter painkiller will help (but please only take as advised by your team and after checking your temperature).

- Changes to eyesight – this is normally temporary and can be frustrating. Please don't rush out and buy new glasses, as your eyesight will normally go back to how it was once chemotherapy finishes. If you need new glasses to see you through treatment, it may be worth getting cheap/temporary ones until your eyesight settles down.

- Diarrhoea/Constipation – this is very common, and you can suffer from both. There are so many different things to try, but your team or GP will advise what's best for you.

- Loss or changes to taste – this can be really distressing, especially if you suddenly can't taste your food, or everything tastes horrible or like cardboard. There really is nothing that can be done to help, and it may only last a few cycles of chemotherapy. It certainly won't be a long-term issue. Unsweetened pineapple juice does seem to help some ladies, and it can be frozen to make a cooling ice lolly as well, but rest assured this is only temporary. The lubricating mouth gel (Biotene) mentioned earlier, may also help with this.

- Nails – Loss or Damage. A very common side effect of chemotherapy is losing nails on your hands and toes. This is because the chemotherapy can react to UV light. If you look at the bags that the drugs come in, you'll notice that some are in a silver pouch to protect it from natural UV light. Although there is no scientific evidence to support this, if you wear a very dark nail varnish (from a few hours before the first chemo straight the way through to several months after treatment ends), it can block the UV from getting to the nails and may prevent you losing them. It doesn't work for everybody, but for the majority, it does. Use any brand you want, but do not use gel nail varnish or any type of false nail that needs to be cured with an LED light. Believe it or not, LEDs contain a small amount of UV, so you could be undoing all the good you're doing. The risk is far less than anything cured with a UV light, but the risk is still there. Also, your nails will be much weaker and putting a false nail on top can make things much worse. For some ladies, wearing dark nail polish doesn't work, but typically they haven't used it all the time. Occasionally nails will be fine during treatment, but then they fall off later, which is why I've suggested you continue to wear the nail polish after treatment ends. There's an alternative that I've heard of but haven't tried myself, and that's to use cuticle oil every day. I don't know how this would work because it doesn't block UV light, but it might afford some protection, and certainly, I know a few ladies who say it's worked for them.

- Cognitive changes to speech, understanding or memory - This is often referred to as "chemo brain", and it's a bit like "baby brain" that women may get after pregnancy. This is normally temporary but can be really worrying as it may affect your day-to-day communication – especially if you're working. Please see the chapter on Cognitive Changes for more information.

- Hand/Foot syndrome – this is normally only associated with Capecitabine, as mentioned earlier, but it can be annoying. Certain creams can help relieve the symptoms and your team or GP will be able to prescribe them.

- Urinary Tract Infections (UTIs) – chemotherapy, and in particular, cyclophosphamide can impact your bladder. This can cause urinary tract infections. If you are uncomfortable and suspect a UTI, speak with your team because they are easy to diagnose and treat with antibiotics. There's no problem taking antibiotics with chemotherapy.

- Thrush – this is another side effect that some ladies suffer with because chemotherapy removes all our good bacteria, as well as the bad. Normally, over the counter tablets and cream will work, but in some cases, thrush can keep returning and be problematic. If this happens, please speak with your team. Sometimes you will be put on a low dose, more frequent treatment, once the initial symptoms are under control. In conjunction with this treatment, you could try a natural alternative. I've found using live, natural yoghurt to be incredibly effective. Dip a tampon into it. Insert the tampon and do this every few hours. The good bacteria in the live yoghurt will help to fight the thrush. I mentioned this in the Facebook group and a lady replied saying that she had sent her husband to buy the yoghurt and he came back with strawberry cheesecake! That definitely wouldn't work, but it did make me chuckle.

Chemotherapy is your friend, not your enemy!

Having just read some of the side effects, you'd be forgiven for being scared about having chemotherapy, but it really is your friend. There are two ways to go into a chemotherapy session:

1. You can go into every chemotherapy session feeling scared (which is normal) and resenting the fact that you have to have chemotherapy. You can hate every minute of it, wish you weren't there and generally wanting to pull the plug and walk away. You might also be frightened of the side effects, and every new ache or pain might worry you.

OR

2. You can go into every chemotherapy session feeling scared but looking at the chemotherapy bags and imagining that it's your own personal army of tiny soldiers going into your body to seek out and destroy the cancer cells. If you watch the infusion, you can use your imagination to see little soldiers

marching into your body. I did this, and honestly, I saw chemotherapy as my lifesaver - my own personal army. And changing my perspective also helped with the side effects. Each time I felt awful (and I did), I would think to myself that if I was feeling terrible, imagine how those tiny cancer cells were feeling being attacked! So, in a way, when I felt at my worst, I hoped that meant that the cancer was being killed off! It did make things a little more bearable, and it was my coping mechanism.

I appreciate that this way of coping with chemotherapy won't work for everybody, but I have found that those ladies who approach everything with a negative mindset will typically have a tougher time getting through treatment. Don't get me wrong. I'm not suggesting you're positive about it (a word I NEVER use with cancer) but finding your inner strength to deal with this new period in your life, is so important.

You will feel awful, you will be exhausted, your body will start to feel like it has a mind of its own, and the side effects can be overwhelming, but this is the same for everybody and must be expected. Of course, there's a limit, and there may be a point where things are unbearable. But for every side effect, there's a pill or a solution, so you mustn't suffer in silence.

It is VERY common to get near to the end of treatment and feel like you can't go on and just want to stop. Again, I would urge you to stick with it. It's a year of your life, and once it's done, it's done. You don't want to give up halfway through and then wish later you'd carried on. I don't say that lightly because I understand completely how chemotherapy can affect you, but please dig deep. I was scheduled for 12 weekly Paclitaxel, but when I got to 8 (and I'd already had 4 x EC also at this point and a break due to illness), I had a meltdown. I didn't feel I could go on, but my oncologist refused to let me stop, and in hindsight, I'm so glad he did. I finished all 12, but it did take a big push from me and a lot of moaning! Find your inner strength if you can.

You must reach out to your team if you're not coping. Sometimes, a simple change of drugs is the answer, but occasionally you may need a break from chemo or new drugs to help. Be realistic though, don't think you're going to be able to function exactly as you did before diagnosis. Be kind to yourself. Your body needs to focus on fighting cancer, and if you're trying to act as normal, you may find it very difficult indeed.

That doesn't mean you should be a couch potato! If you feel like gentle exercising, do it. It's good to keep as active as you can during treatment but don't push yourself.

What to Wear On the Day of Chemotherapy

Wear comfortable clothes, and don't forget that your team will need access to your Port or PICC line (if you have one), so don't wear restrictive clothing that would make that difficult. If you're going to be examined, easy clothes to get on and off is also sensible.

Travelling To Your Chemotherapy Session

It is always recommended that you get somebody to take you both to and from your chemotherapy treatments and you don't drive yourself. Some chemotherapy treatments have alcohol in them and maybe enough to put you over the limit. If you were to drive after chemotherapy and have an accident, your insurance might be void.

If you are struggling to get to your appointments, please speak with your team. Some hospitals can provide transportation, but it does need to be pre-booked.

What to Take On the Day of Chemotherapy

Lots of ladies get very worried about how to prepare for chemotherapy and what to take on the day. I often look back and laugh at what happened to me. I asked everybody what I needed and then dutifully bought everything that was suggested and turned up at my first chemotherapy appointment…… with a suitcase! Yes, I was that person! Subsequent chemotherapies, I was better prepared, with just a handbag! However, there are some items that make sense to take:

- If you've been given a chemotherapy record book (not everybody gets one), you need to have that with you because the nurses may update it every cycle.

- If you want to use your phone, a charger with a long lead is a good idea in case there are delays, and you'll be at the hospital for longer than normal.

- A book, magazine or kindle might be something to keep you occupied.

- I know some ladies take bottled water or sweets and even something to eat, but that's really personal preference and depends on the time you're going in. Don't forget if you need food or drink; your hospital may be able to help with that anyway.

- If you are cold capping, you may want to take some additional warm clothes to wear during the session (so perhaps a bigger bag than your normal handbag), and definitely a warm head covering, as you will probably be leaving the hospital with wet hair. Blankets etc. will be given to you by the hospital, so don't bother with them unless you have a favourite one and would prefer to take your own with you.

What to Eat/Avoid During Chemotherapy

This is a strange topic because there doesn't seem to be an agreed consensus between oncologists, which isn't very helpful! Some ladies are told to eat as if they're pregnant, so avoid anything unpasteurised, take-aways, raw and undercooked meat, raw or uncooked eggs etc. The basis of this is that these foods might cause certain bacteria to grow and as you're immunosuppressed, you could become ill.

However, the majority of oncologists give no diet advice at all! I wasn't given any advice other than to eat as healthily as I could, but to eat what I wanted, especially if my taste was affected. Listen to your team and decide what's best for you.

Alcohol, though, may become a problem! For some reason, when you're having treatment, your tolerance to alcohol might be non-existent and having one drink might get you dancing on tables! Again, take advice from your oncologist, but an occasional drink is usually permitted!

Sex and Cancer Treatments

For anybody sexually active going through cancer treatments, life can continue as normal, or it may affect how you feel about being intimate with a partner. Chemotherapy can reduce your sexual desires and of course, how you're feeling emotionally will play a big part too. If you're concerned, it's worth talking to your team or GP, but don't put yourself under pressure. There are only a few pieces of advice I would give, and that is, if your partner is male, he should be encouraged to wear a condom. If you're having chemotherapy, there is a slim chance of it transferring to him and clearly, that's not what you want. The risk is at its highest in the first few days after chemotherapy, but it's sensible to take precautions throughout treatment, rather than just the first few days.

Exciting Treatment Advances:

Pembrolizumab (Keytruda) Immunotherapy

In 2017, a Phase III drug trial, KEYNOTE 522, evaluated the use of an immunotherapy drug, Pembrolizumab (Trade name Keytruda), given alongside chemotherapy for the treatment of early locally advanced Triple-Negative breast cancer (stages 1c, 2 and 3). The trial was successful in demonstrating, when compared with a group who had a placebo/chemotherapy, patients that had Pembrolizumab/chemotherapy had better overall outcomes in two areas, namely (1) achieved a complete pathological response (i.e., no cancer in the breast, nodes, or skin) after treatment, and (2) the longer-term recurrence rate was lower. Please read the next chapter on immunotherapy for more information.

Accordingly, NICE is currently considering whether to authorise its use for early locally advanced Triple Negative breast cancer in England (and, presumably, this will filter to Scotland, Wales, and Ireland). This is not guaranteed, but in the anticipation that it may be used for primary Triple Negative breast cancer, it's worth expanding on how it may be used. The treatment regime, if it follows the trial, is likely to be:

1. Pembrolizumab (once every three weeks) to be given with Paclitaxel (weekly) and Carboplatin (weekly or once every three weeks) for four cycles (i.e., 12 weeks)

2. Pembrolizumab (once every three weeks) to be given with Epirubicin plus Cyclophosphamide (EC) OR Adriamycin plus Cyclophosphamide (AC) (once every three weeks) for four cycles (i.e., 12 weeks)

3. Surgery (lumpectomy or mastectomy with sentinel or axillary node removal) 3-6 weeks after (2) above

4. Radiotherapy if required

5. Pembrolizumab (once every three weeks) for nine cycles (i.e., 27 weeks)

The trial was licenced to include stages 1c (tumour is more than 1cm but not more than 2cm) <u>with</u> 1-2 nodes involved OR stage 2 or 3 with 0-2 (or more) nodes involved. It is likely that these will be the same parameters for offering Pembrolizumab to patients once licenced by NICE. This does mean, if your tumour is 2cm or less but you don't have affected nodes, you wouldn't qualify for this treatment.

Additionally, the trial included patients who were both PDL1 positive AND negative, so it's likely that this may not be a factor when deciding who can have the treatment, which is excellent as it opens the door to many more patients. For more information on PDL1 status, please see the next chapter on immunotherapy. If timelines follow the drug trial, they are likely to be as follows, and will be longer than the typical chemotherapy regimes in use now:

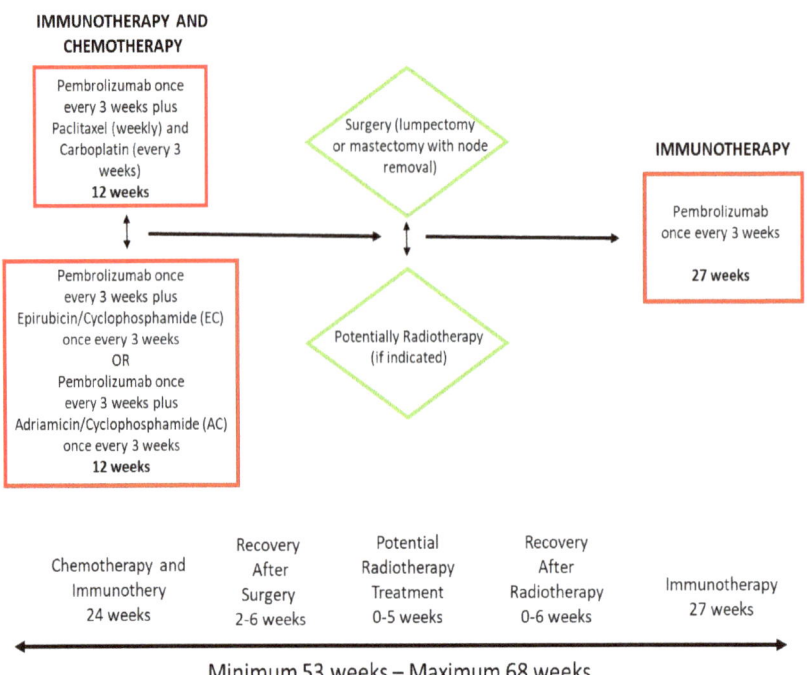

IMMUNOTHERAPY AND CHEMOTHERAPY

Pembrolizumab once every 3 weeks plus Paclitaxel (weekly) and Carboplatin (every 3 weeks)
12 weeks

Pembrolizumab once every 3 weeks plus Epirubicin/Cyclophosphamide (EC) once every 3 weeks
OR
Pembrolizumab once every 3 weeks plus Adriamicin/Cyclophosphamide (AC) once every 3 weeks
12 weeks

Surgery (lumpectomy or mastectomy with node removal)

Potentially Radiotherapy (if indicated)

IMMUNOTHERAPY

Pembrolizumab once every 3 weeks

27 weeks

Chemotherapy and Immunothery
24 weeks

Recovery After Surgery
2-6 weeks

Potential Radiotherapy Treatment
0-5 weeks

Recovery After Radiotherapy
0-6 weeks

Immunotherapy
27 weeks

Minimum 53 weeks – Maximum 68 weeks
(assuming no delays)

CHAPTER 14

IMMUNOTHERAPY

Immunotherapy isn't a new form of treatment, but until the past five years or so, it wasn't used for breast cancer, but was more commonly used to treat lung, brain, bladder cancers etc. The reason is that certain treatments don't work with all types of cancer, and to ensure its effectiveness, trials must take place.

For immunotherapy with breast cancer, the trials began with people who had Stage 4 breast cancers and then moved to early breast cancer. After the trials, certain immunotherapy drugs were licenced for use with stage 4 breast cancer, and as mentioned earlier, approval is in the late stages for use with early breast cancers.

Now for the bad news – unfortunately, immunotherapy doesn't work for every Triple Negative breast cancer, AND it's also shown to be most effective when it's combined with chemotherapy. So, unfortunately, it doesn't replace chemotherapy. Why doesn't it work for all people? Let's take a look at how it works.

Immunotherapy targets cancer cells differently from chemotherapy. Chemotherapy looks for predominately misshapen cells, but it can't recognise healthy cells – so it kills everything in its path. With immunotherapy, the drug targets your immune system, turning it on, so it recognises an invader and allows it to attack the cancer cells - so healthy cells are left alone.

With immunotherapy, our immune system is the key to killing cancer cells, but the problem is that the immune system actually has to "see" the cells for it to target the cancer. Think about your immune system like this - it recognises good cells that are part of you and does nothing because it likes them. However, if it detects a harmful cell, the immune system is stimulated to fight – just like when you have a cold or virus. Now, this is where the problem starts! Cancer can be tricky and doesn't always like to be seen, and as it grows, it can develop ways to hide from the immune system. When it does this, the cancer can grow and spread without the immune system seeing it or kicking in. Cancer uses different ways to disguise itself from the immune system, which is why one immunotherapy may work for patient A but be useless for patient B (both of whom have Triple Negative) because the cancer is using a different shield.

The aim of immunotherapy is to detect how the cancer hides, turn off the shields and allow the immune system to see the cells and send treatment to kill them.

So how do we know if immunotherapy may work for us? In our bodies, we have a protein called PDL1 (Programmed Death Ligand 1). PDL1 is a protein that helps keep immune cells from attacking good cells in the body. Some cancer cells have high amounts of PDL1 (you would be told you are PDL1 positive if this is the case). However, high levels of PDL1, allow cancer cells to "trick" the immune system, and avoid being attacked as foreign, harmful substances. Immunotherapy therefore targets PDL1 to turn it off, so the cancer cells are seen. Unfortunately, not everybody has a high level of PDL1, and without this, immunotherapy may not work as the cancer shield may not turn off.

To determine your levels of PDL1, a simple blood test or biopsy will be carried out. For those who are PDL1 positive, immunotherapy is more likely to work, although not guaranteed (even with high levels of PDL1). For those who are PDL1 negative, immunotherapy may or may not work. In America, immunotherapy has been given to PDL1 negative Triple Negative breast cancer patients, and in some cases, it does seem to have an effect. This is encouraging, and certainly, a 2017 trial looking at combining Pembrolizumab (immunotherapy) with chemotherapy for early breast cancers, was given to patients who were both PDL1 positive and negative. This is the immunotherapy that will hopefully be licenced for use in England in late 2022 for early locally advanced Triple Negative breast cancer.

Side effects, like with chemotherapy, can be tough. All the typical side effects with chemotherapy are similar to immunotherapy, so this treatment is not without its own sets of challenges, and don't forget, you are likely to have both together.

Immunotherapy is very exciting, and I'm sure that in another 10-20 years, there will be even more developments.

CHAPTER 15

SURGERY

This chapter focuses on breast surgery in general, but if you would like to understand the different types of reconstruction (if having a mastectomy), they are covered in the next chapter.

Prior to being diagnosed, if somebody had said "lumpectomy" or "mastectomy" to me, it would have conjured up an image of hideously scarred breasts, but this is absolutely not true. Whatever surgery you have, breasts may look a bit different than before but, there's no reason, unless you want to tell someone, that they would ever know. Scars fade over time, and for some ladies, they fade to the point where they are incredibly difficult to see. Even ladies who chose to have a mastectomy and remain flat, without reconstruction, can have very neat scars and it's only without clothes that anybody would know they'd had surgery.

For many ladies with Triple Negative breast cancer, a lumpectomy is the preferred surgery because it's far less invasive, keeps all feeling in the breast area, and will be appropriate for around 60-70% of patients.

There are photographs online of all different end results, but the best measure is to ask your surgeon to show you photos of their work. They will also be able to tell you exactly what's possible in your individual case, where scars may be positioned and what result may be achieved.

Different Main Types of Surgery:

Lumpectomy (Wide Local Excision - WLE)

And

Mastectomy

Which one will you have? It's typically a discussion between you and your surgeon. Sometimes, they will suggest one may be better than the other. There are no rights or wrongs, and both will remove cancer, so there isn't really a "better" surgery. That said, there are some differences that are worth discussing, so you can have a consultation with your surgeon after thinking through all the options.

Statistically, having a lumpectomy or mastectomy gives you the same percentage of surviving your CURRENT breast cancer. Why? Well, they both take away the affected breast tissue. What NEITHER do, is remove the risk of spread if cells have escaped, and the chemotherapy/radiotherapy hasn't zapped them. So, you'd wonder why anybody would have a mastectomy if the percentages were the same? Well, there are two reasons.

1. If you carry a defective gene, i.e., BRCA1, BRCA2, PALB2, ATM, CHEK2, to name a few, your chances of getting another breast cancer (in the same or opposite breast) increases. Having a mastectomy (and usually a double if you have the defective gene), decreases the risk of another breast cancer or recurrence to the breast (there are a few exceptions

to this mentioned below). However, when you are first diagnosed, you may not know whether you're a carrier of the defective gene. This test can take a few months to get the result, so you may have a lumpectomy or a single mastectomy, but later, when the results are back, you will probably be offered a double mastectomy (or single mastectomy to the remaining breast).

2. With Triple Negative, the risk of recurrence, or a new breast cancer, in either your bad breast, or the good one, increases to around 25% (an average of the statistics found online), whether you have nodes involved or not. So, would you be reducing your risk of a recurrence/new breast cancer if you had a mastectomy? Certainly, there's less breast tissue for a recurrence to come back to, but there are no guarantees.

There are also reasons why you may be urged to have a lumpectomy over a mastectomy. For example, if your tumour is close to the chest wall, it may be advised not to have a mastectomy. The reason is that if the breast tissue is removed, there is a risk, if the cancer were to come back, it would come back in a similar place, and without having breast tissue, it could (not always) go to the chest wall or the scar area where it would be more problematic to treat. Your surgeon will be able to tell you if your tumour is near to the chest wall.

Surgeons tend to favour a lumpectomy wherever possible because it's a smaller operation, preserves the breast, and if you have clear nodes, there's every indication that surgery will remove the cancer successfully, and you will not require any other surgery.

Lumpectomy – Wide Local Excision

So, let's look a bit more at the lumpectomy option. You may be offered a lumpectomy (WLE) if your cancer can be removed, leaving your breast intact. Your tumour (either before or after chemotherapy), needs to be small in comparison to your breast size so it can be removed, and your breast retains its shape. This is called breast-conserving surgery, and where possible, offered to a patient. Keeping your breast may be very important to you, and with a lumpectomy, it will be a minimally invasive surgery, with a faster recovery. This can be easier, both mentally and physically, to deal with.

Let's explore this surgery a little further. A lumpectomy is where a "lump" or tumour area, is removed together with some surrounding tissue. Why take surrounding tissue? Well, tumour cells can grow and move and sometimes, as they grow, they will start to infiltrate the area surrounding the tumour. It's extremely important to remove these cells, which are small and normally won't be seen on a scan.

The only time these cells are detected is when the removed tissue goes to the laboratory and is examined using high magnification. The surgeon's aim is to make sure that, after surgery, you are free of cancer. That means there must be an area surrounding the tumour that is free of cancer cells, called "clear margins". Surprisingly, the margins only need to be 1mm (all around the tumour). That sounds like a tiny margin but think how tiny the cells are – 1mm is actually huge by comparison.

What happens if the margins are not clear and the laboratory reports there are cancer cells within the 1mm edge? Typically, the surgeon will then operate again and "shave" the cavity to remove another layer of tissue where the tumour has been. Unfortunately, the surgeon is working blind because they can't "see" the cells, so they take what they think is appropriate. Rarely, but it does happen, a surgeon may not achieve clear margins a second time, and at that point, the decision will be either, do another cavity shave, OR change the type of surgery to a mastectomy, to ensure all affected cells are removed.

At the same time, when removing the tumour and surrounding area, the surgeon will normally remove nodes as well. Even if scans have shown the nodes are free of cancer, the surgeon will probably take a few sentinel nodes so the laboratory can check for microscopic cells (again, these are unlikely to show on scans).

The number of nodes removed will depend on what has shown in your scans beforehand. If the scans have shown a high uptake of cancer cells, the surgeon will take what they think is appropriate, and in some cases, it could involve removing all nodes in the armpit.

What Will My Scars Be Like?

Typically, with a lumpectomy, your scar will be a few inches long, but of course, this depends on the size and position of your tumour. As a lumpectomy is normally performed on smaller tumours (or tumours that have been shrunk by chemotherapy), the scar is not very big and a thin line that will fade over time. The node removal scar is also typically around a few inches long and will be somewhere near the armpit. Occasionally if the tumour is near to the nodes, you may only have one scar, which of course, is a bonus.

Will a Lumpectomy Change How My Breast Looks?

Apart from the scar, in most cases, there will be no other change to the way your breast looks compared to before breast cancer. Very occasionally, there may be a dent where the tumour has been removed, but your surgeon has lots of ways to rectify this, for example, lipo modelling, sculpting, filling and even breast lifts, reductions, mammoplasties, and perforator flaps. So, there's usually a solution.

A lumpectomy will retain your breast's natural appearance, and will resemble your breast before cancer, much more so than a mastectomy, which may change the way the breast(s) look. If symmetry is important, it's usually easier to achieve with a lumpectomy.

What Are the Advantages of a Lumpectomy?

Here are just a few:

- You keep your breast.

- You retain all feeling in your breast and nipple area – this is hugely important to some ladies and should be taken into consideration.

- The breast may look exactly like your other breast, because of the less invasive surgery.

- Surveillance to check for any issues in the breast area in the future can include mammograms (you can't have these with certain mastectomies – depending on the reconstruction). This can be a HUGE consideration for ladies who want to be able to have easier check-ups moving forward.

- There's less downtime after surgery, and recovery is normally quicker than a mastectomy.

- Psychologically it may be easier to deal with.

What Is Surgery Like for a Lumpectomy?

The order of what happens and what you have done will differ depending on your surgeon and the hospital. Here are a few of the steps that may happen (in any order):

When you had your tumour biopsied, you may have had a marker or Magseed inserted. This can be done at any time but is usually, with the help of an ultrasound, to mark the exact spot of your tumour at first diagnosis. Markers are normally the size of a metal sesame seed, and they help to guide the surgeon to the right spot. They are also useful because they show up on scans, so if you're having chemotherapy before surgery and your tumour melts away, the marker remains, so the surgeon knows the area to remove. Typically, you just have one marker, but occasionally you may have more.

At the time of writing, there are a couple of types of markers. Some are just markers that will show up on scans, but the more modern type (Magseeds), includes a tiny amount of radioactivity, and the surgeon can track the marker with a specialist tool during surgery. The new markers sometimes (but not always) eliminate the need for guide wires.

Guide wires! Well, this was a shock to me because I had no idea that anything like this was going to be needed. A guide wire does exactly what it says on the tin! It points to the tumour area to help the surgeon during surgery. They are only inserted on the day, or sometimes the day before, surgery. The guide wire itself is about 1mm across (possibly less), but on the end that goes into the breast, it has little prongs to keep it in place so it can't fall out (which is why you should never try to pull it out – not that I'm sure you would)!

To insert the guide wire, your breast will be numbed using a cream or spray, and you'll feel a bit of pressure as it's inserted. This feels similar to the biopsies you've had, and you hear a click (like a stapler) as it goes in. It's mildly uncomfortable but definitely tolerable. The radiographer will then check that the guide wire is in place using an ultrasound machine and then a mammogram. If you're unlucky like me, and it's not in the right place, you may need a second one put in!

You may also have a colourless and/or blue radioactive dye injected into your breast either before or during surgery. This is done with the help of a scanning machine, and you are scanned first, then injected with the dye (with a local anaesthetic), and you may be asked to get off the bed and walk around and massage your breast a bit. This is to encourage the dye to move around the breast.

During surgery, your surgeon will look at this dye using a special tool to illuminate the path from the tumour to the sentinel nodes and beyond. This helps the surgeon decide which nodes to remove (not all nodes will be in the path from the tumour to the nodes, so they may not be removed). If the radioactive blue dye is used (and this might even be administered during surgery rather than before), it has a peculiar side effect that you may have a patch of electric blue skin which can take months to fade! I was strangely attached to mine and was upset when it disappeared! I liked looking like a Smurf!

To protect your breasts after surgery, you will probably be asked to wear a front fastening, non-wired bra for 4-6 weeks 24/7. This holds the breast firmly so that where the lump has been removed, it doesn't have too much movement and encourages healing. You should get a bra that's your normal size or one back size larger, especially because you'll be wearing it in bed, and as our size can fluctuate during the day, it may be more comfortable to wear a bra that isn't too tight.

What you may find is that the bra under your arm will hit the spot of your lymph node removal scar (or if your tumour is low on your breast, then by the crease on the underside). To stop this rubbing and hampering healing, ask your breast care nurse for some soft gauze and tuck that under any seams that are hurting.

The tissue removed at surgery, will be sent to the laboratory for analysis, and you will have a meeting with the surgeon a few weeks later to discuss the results.

Mastectomy

A mastectomy can be considered for any size of breast cancer, and you may be offered this even if your tumour is very small. However, it is commonly suggested to ladies who either have a defective gene, a large tumour, or have node involvement. There's no one rule that fits everybody because, for example, you may have a really large tumour at diagnosis, but then have chemotherapy, and by the time you get to surgery, the tumour has shrunk so much that a lumpectomy can be considered.

With a mastectomy, which of course if a much larger operation, there are different options such as staying flat, or having an immediate or delayed reconstruction. It's not always possible to have what you want and occasionally, for example, an immediate reconstruction cannot be considered, but you may be offered a delayed reconstruction. There are usually solutions for everything, but I'd urge you to work with your surgeon to find one that's right for you if a mastectomy is being considered.

If you are thinking of having a reconstruction, not all surgeons perform all types of reconstruction, so you may be referred to specialists to determine whether you may be suitable. Different reconstructions depend on certain criteria, so this will also be a determining factor in your suitability. It can be very useful to meet with different surgeons to go through all options, as it may also highlight different reconstructions you may not have considered. It may also help you to come to terms with what you can realistically achieve, and what won't be possible.

Surgery for a mastectomy can take anywhere from 4-12 hours (depending on whether there's a reconstruction or not). The aim is to take away most of the breast tissue from either one or both breasts, including the nipple area. Scars are very much dependent on your surgeon and type of reconstruction (if any). Once removed, the tissue is analysed by the laboratory, and you'll have a meeting with your surgeon (normally two weeks after surgery) to go through the results.

Recovery from a mastectomy will take longer than a lumpectomy because it is a larger operation with bigger scars. However, the recovery process is similar to a lumpectomy. You will need to sleep upright for a few weeks, and if you've had a reconstruction, you will need to wear a supportive bra (and potentially other supports – depending on the reconstruction) day and night for 4 or more weeks.

With a mastectomy, it's common to have temporary "drains" put in during surgery to remove excess fluid and allow your body to heal. The drain consists of a very thin tube that comes out of the side of the breast (if in that area), down to a collecting chamber that fills up during the day. Drains need to be kept lower than your breast area to allow for the fluid to react with gravity. Sleeping upright helps with this.

The number of drains you have, depends on whether you're having a single or double mastectomy and type of reconstruction. For example, if you're having a double mastectomy with implant reconstruction, you'll probably only have a drain to each mastectomy side. With a double DIEP reconstruction, you may have a drain on each side for the breasts, and then one on either side of your tummy, so a total of 4.

You'll be taught how to empty and record the amount of fluid every day. This gives your surgeon an indication how well you're healing. Not all surgeons use drains, and honestly, they can be a bit of a nuisance, but they really do work, so don't be scared of them. Normally they stay in for 1-2 weeks, and you'll be given drain bags to keep them in, if you need to go out, for example.

Removal of the drains is easy – you take a deep breath in, and they are pulled out within seconds. It doesn't hurt and is just a bit of pulling. In fact, it's an odd feeling, and I was terrified of having it done but was really surprised at how easy it was.

No Reconstruction after Surgery

For some ladies, the thought of having a reconstruction is not even a consideration. They've been through so much and are happy to stay flat. There's absolutely nothing to say that ladies must have a reconstruction, and for some, remaining flat is a liberation. I've seen some fantastic photos of ladies who have remained flat and have had tattoos that cover the breast area. For me, this wasn't a consideration, but it's wholly appropriate for many ladies, and I celebrate their decision.

If you're considering this route, I would strongly suggest joining the "Flat Friends" Facebook group and chatting with others. They will give you the best advice, and if you feel that staying flat in a bikini, for example, might be problematic, the group will be able to help with lots of ideas. There are lots of companies that offer prosthetics and/or lingerie that includes inserts if you want to try them, so there's no reason for you to feel self-conscious. Honestly, I've seen ladies, after remaining flat, who wear gorgeous bralettes and bikinis and you'd never know they had had major surgery.

Some ladies find that after being flat for a while, they miss their breasts and want a shapelier figure. In some cases, it may be possible, but it can present a challenge – for example, the original mastectomy scars may not be placed in the right area, you may not have enough remaining skin etc., therefore your reconstruction options may be limited. However, everything is possible, but you may need to find a surgeon who can assess your case and advise accordingly.

General Surgery Information

What to Take on the Day of Surgery

Surgery, for either a lumpectomy or mastectomy, can either be as a day case, overnight or several nights, so what you take with you depends on the length of stay. To help your thought process, I would suggest:

- Easy to put on pyjamas and a dressing gown. A button-front pair of pyjamas is easier, especially if you're staying in hospital and likely to have doctors popping in to see how you're doing and check dressings etc. I prefer a longer type dressing gown because if you're wearing one of the hospital gowns, they can put your bum on display and are impossible to tie without being a contortionist, so a longer dressing gown protects your modesty!

- Slippers – you'll need these to walk to the theatre.

- Although you may not need your post-surgery bra straight after surgery, it might be worth taking with you just in case.

- Any medications you're taking together with your chemotherapy record book if you have one at that stage.

- A phone charger and long lead if you want to use your phone

- A book or kindle to keep you amused.

- Toiletries and I would definitely include a packet of wet wipes. These are fantastic if you just want a bit of a refresh at any point. They are my "go-to" in my hospital bag.

- Comfortable clothes to go home in. To give you less packing, wear these clothes to go into hospital as well. Choose a top that doesn't require you to lift your arms up. A button or front fastening zip-top is the best. Also, think about your shoes – easy to slip on shoes or boots are much easier than something you must lace up!

- Glasses if you need them. You may have to read and sign forms.

- Socks – if your feet get cold, having a pair of socks should keep you cosy.

You will be asked to remove ALL jewellery, although they usually allow you to keep your wedding band if you wear one. I take all mine off and leave it at home as it's just easier.

If you have false nails or are wearing nail polish, these need to be removed. The reason behind this is that your nails can be an indicator of oxygen levels and blood circulation during surgery and having anything on your nails can impede that. I was told of a lady who was admitted to hospital for surgery but was wearing gel nails, and the hospital went into a panic because they couldn't remove them. They had to send out a note to all nurses reminding them to tell patients to remove false nails before surgery!

Although you will be given a time when you must stop eating and drinking, please make sure the day before you are admitted, you drink as much water as you can to stay hydrated. This will help your veins be more prominent, which is always a bonus when you're having bloods taken and an anaesthetic.

Surgery Complications

Sadly, surgery complications do occur. Very rarely are they long term, and typically they are short term, but can be a worry when they happen to you. Here are a few of the more common issues:

Seroma

A seroma, which is a localised build-up of fluid, usually presents itself around 5-10 days after surgery. You may feel a sloshing sensation (as if there's fluid in the breast). This is exactly what it is, and accompanying this, the skin may also be red and feel hot and may become infected. If drains are used after surgery, as mentioned above, seromas are often dealt with by them. However, drains are not commonly used with a lumpectomy and are more common with mastectomy surgeries.

A seroma can stop the surrounding area from healing, but once it's under control, the healing process will continue. Normally, seromas are reabsorbed back into the body within a few weeks, but in some cases, they need to be drained manually if a drain has not been used, which will give immediate relief. Manual draining is usually done by inserting a very thin needle and drawing off the fluid. Occasionally, it may need draining more than once over the course of a few weeks. If the liquid isn't clear, you may be given antibiotics to combat any infection. A seroma, whilst very uncomfortable, does normally resolve with some help, but the area may be slightly scared, and subsequent scans may spot this even a few years after it's resolved.

Lymphoedema

Lymphoedema can occur to the cancer side arm after surgery or radiotherapy but very occasionally will be present in the breast, too, although this is much rarer. The lymphatic system is designed to move and drain fluid around the body, and if lymph nodes are removed, this can interfere with the process. Having a few sentinel nodes removed is less likely to expose you to lymphoedema as the remaining nodes will continue to do their intended job. However, if you have multiple nodes, or full node removal, you are more at risk.

Lymphoedema can start at any time and may begin without warning. It can also be triggered if you have an infection in that arm, a bite from an insect, a cut, exposure to heat and sunburn etc., so you should protect your arm wherever possible. If anything happens that breaks the skin on that arm, wash and disinfect the area immediately.

You'll also probably be told that having any blood tests, blood pressure, or anything done to that arm is a complete no-no. Current guidelines seem to indicate that it may be safe to take blood out but not put anything into the arm, but each hospital, and oncologist, has their own thoughts on this. Please speak with your team for their advice, but if in doubt, good practice is to avoid using your node removal arm wherever possible.

There's an easy trick to check to see if you have lymphoedema – get some bubble wrap or something similar that has bumps. Tuck it into your bra or inside your sleeve around your arm for an hour or so. If you can do it on your good and bad sides, it will be easier to compare results. If it's lymphoedema, the bubble wrap will leave indents in your skin that take longer to disappear than your good side. Of course, this test is not fool proof, but it gives you an idea if there's a fluid build-up.

Lymphoedema can be really painful as the arm (or part of it), will swell and look puffy, which is because the fluid is struggling to drain away. If it becomes a longer-term problem, compression garments are usually worn to help, and it may be that you must wear them 24/7. There are also exercises that encourage drainage, and specialised massages called manual lymphatic drainage may be offered. It's important to ask for a referral to your hospital's lymphoedema clinic as they have experts who can help with your symptoms and can teach you the correct way to help drainage.

Necrosis

With any type of surgery, necrosis (dead tissue) can happen. Necrosis is when a patch of tissue dies, normally because of a lack of blood supply. This can happen internally or externally. Externally, it typically presents as a blackened area, so it's easy to spot. If necrosis is external, it will be removed unless it's very small and in which case your surgeon may just monitor it, until they feel it should be removed – sometimes, it's best to let things settle down before intervening, especially if the area is small. If the necrosis is large and external, it can be problematic if you've had a reconstruction because this may mean that after removal, your breast will be smaller than before. Of course, in many cases, size can be adjusted later.

Internal necrosis can either be removed surgically or left alone, depending on what has caused it, but it may show on any future scan if left in the breast. If you are having a scan after all treatment has ended, it's worth mentioning to the scan team so they're aware.

Aching, Numbness, Tingling and Shooting Pains

With any breast surgery, nerves and blood vessels must be cut, and this is unavoidable. This can cause numbness and tingling, and as everything knits back together, it can also cause sharp shooting pains, a bit like an electric shock. This is nothing to worry about, and actually, the pains can be reassuring because it can indicate you're healing. Feelings should come back to numb areas, but this can take a while. If it's not tolerable, you may be referred to physiotherapy to try to encourage healing.

During chemotherapy, you may also have an ache or pain in the tumour area – this can be a sign that chemotherapy is getting to work on that area and is very common but worrying if you're not sure why it's happening. My oncologist told me that if you have a "weak" area, for example, an area where surgery has been performed or from an earlier accident etc., the aching feeling is common in that spot. I liked to feel the ache where my tumour had been because it reassured me the chemotherapy was getting to work. Not everybody will feel this, so please don't worry if you don't.

Pulmonary Embolism (PE)

As with any surgery, a pulmonary embolism (blood clot) can develop, and it's also a side effect of chemotherapy as well. A clot can present itself in different ways:

- Pain, tightness, redness/discolouration, heat and swelling typically of the calf, leg, or thigh or over a vein OR it can be near to, or by, your PICC or Port line. It may also present itself in the arm, chest, or neck area.

- Shortness of breath may be sudden or increases over time

- Pain or tightness in the chest area when you take a deep breath or cough

- You may also have an unexplained cough (may cough up blood)

If you experience any of these symptoms either after surgery, or during chemotherapy, please reach out to your team immediately. A blood test, scans and examination are usually sufficient to be able to diagnose a blood clot. Treatment is with the use of a blood thinner – either injections or tablets and your treatment may be paused for a short time to allow the drugs to work. Please don't worry if this happens to you. Blood clots are a common side effect, but they do need immediate intervention. If you suspect you have one, please get in touch with your team quickly.

New Lumps or Bumps

With any breast surgery, because your breast tissue and node area have been moved around, it can cause scar tissue, adhesions, or necrosis in certain areas. These often present as a new lump and can be really worrying, but they are normally left alone and will become the new you. However, for peace of mind, it is always wise to get these checked. New lumps, that are on your scar line, or near the site of your tumour, are definitely ones to be checked, because if cancer is going to return, it can come back to the original site (not always, so please don't panic). The majority of new lumps are really nothing to worry about. I can't tell you the number of panicked women I've seen over the years who spend a few weeks of hell after discovering a new lump, worrying as to what it may be. These lumps and bumps, once you've been reassured they're nothing to be concerned about, will become your new normal, and are unlikely to disappear.

Ongoing Pain in the Breast Area

Unfortunately, and especially with a reconstruction, there can be ongoing pain issues. Normally these are mild and don't interfere with everyday life and are just your body readjusting. However, in a small percentage of cases, pain can be scar tissue and adhesions that "stick" areas together that normally wouldn't be attached. This means as you move around, the areas feel tight and can be painful.

Further surgery can remove and cut through these adhesions to free up the area and give you back movement. Just bear in mind that each surgery has the potential to cause adhesions and can happen again, so it's worth chatting through the options with your surgeon.

Cording after Node Removal

Cording, as the name suggests, is when muscles and veins can harden and feel like cords under the skin. It can affect normal movement and be painful when the arm is stretched. Thankfully this is normally short term and can be helped with heat and gentle massage. Massage needs to be applied correctly, so it's a good idea to see a physiotherapist who can teach you the correct technique. Your team should be able to refer you to the hospital's physio team.

CHAPTER 16

DIFFERENT TYPES OF BREAST RECONSTRUCTION

There are two main types of reconstruction (1) implants and (2) autologous or "flap" reconstruction. A "flap" reconstruction, in very basic terms, uses a selection of either fat, muscles or blood vessels, from other areas of your body, to create a new breast. Although there are quite a few types of flap reconstruction, I've only listed the more readily available surgeries in the UK at the present time. Most of these procedures are carried out by highly skilled specialist consultants, and you may have to travel to a different hospital where they have the facilities to carry out these surgeries if not offered at your hospital:

- Deep Inferior Epigastric Perforators (DIEP)
- Latissimus Dorsi (LD)
- Transverse Upper Gracilis (TUG)
- Transverse Rectus Abdominis (TRAM)
- Gluteal Artery Perforator (IGAP or SGAP)

Implant Reconstruction

Implants are the "easiest" type of reconstruction for a patient, and you may need just one operation. However, if you're having radiotherapy, you may find that a reconstruction using implants isn't recommended or poses some challenges. This is because radiotherapy can cause your skin to change, and the changes may continue for several years. Typically, the skin thickens and loses its elasticity. Implants don't like radiotherapy, and it can cause irreparable damage to the implant itself. The implant could encapsulate – the thing you don't want with an implant. There are ways around this, and it may be worth asking your surgeon if any of these options would work for you:

1. You could ask if there would be an option to have a temporary expander put in to hold the skin in place. Once the skin has settled down, the expander is removed and replaced with an implant. An expander allows you to have the shape of a breast after surgery. However, expanders can be uncomfortable.

2. You could ask if there's a possibility of having a temporary implant, just for radiotherapy, that is swapped out at a later date.

These solutions may not be appropriate, but if you want implants, this may be something to ask about.

There are also choices to be made with an implant reconstruction. The implant can be placed over the muscle or under the muscle and you may also be able to choose the shape of the implant (typically round or teardrop). In some cases, your surgeon will also talk to you about the types of mesh used to create the sling that the implant sits in.

There's no right and wrong decision here. Implants under the muscle can give a more natural appearance as you won't see the shape of the implant. Over the muscle, the implant shape may be more obvious, but the procedure doesn't move the muscle, so recovery is usually easier. If you exercise a lot, this may be a consideration because as you exercise, the pectoral muscles move and can squeeze the implant causing (over time) some change to the shape.

In terms of the shape of the implants, a round implant is more obvious and less natural-looking than a teardrop shape. However, it's important to speak with your surgeon about the likely end result they will be able to achieve in your case.

Unlike a boob job, implants with a mastectomy do not give a typical projection, and from the side, your breasts can have a slightly flatter look. This is not noticeable when wearing clothes, but you may notice it when naked (although it's highly unlikely anybody but you would be aware of it).

The size of implants can be discussed with your surgeon, but typically they don't like to commit beforehand by saying, "you'll be an X cup", for example. A good surgeon will determine the size of the implant based on your frame, and also on what is achievable with the skin that is left from the mastectomy. Therefore, if you want to be a specific size and shape, implants may not be for you.

A few things you need to be aware of is that lying on your tummy might be problematic. I don't know if ladies who just have a boob job have this problem, but with implant reconstruction, it can be uncomfortable lying on your tummy.

Also, and this is very weird, the implants can feel cold even though they don't make you feel cold! I don't know how to describe this because it's so odd, but I can feel a perfect temperature, but then I put my hands on my breasts, and they feel cold! They never make me feel cold, though, so it's only if you touch your breasts that you'll notice it. It's a very strange sensation, but you only notice it if you actively think about it!

DIEP Reconstruction

At the time of writing, a DIEP reconstruction is considered to be the gold standard of reconstruction. A DIEP takes tummy fat to create either one or two new breasts. In effect, it's using your own body tissue, which is always an advantage as it reduces the risk of your body rejecting foreign tissue.

However, not everybody will be a candidate. For this operation, you need sufficient tummy fat to recreate either one or both breasts. Also, you need to have very good veins in your lower tummy area as these are removed and repositioned in the breast to ensure a good blood supply to your new breasts. Not everybody can fulfil this criterion, but most do.

I very much wanted a DIEP, but unfortunately, after seeing three consultants, I was told I didn't have enough fat/tissue to recreate two nice size breasts that would suit my frame. I was devastated, but one surgeon told me to have implants and, if I didn't get on with them, to see her again and potentially I could have a DIEP with either smaller breasts or with the addition of implants, at a later date. I very much liked this approach but, in the end, opted for implants and, for me, that was the correct decision.

In terms of surgery and recovery time, a DIEP is a long process and can take around 9-12 hours in surgery. It usually involves two surgeons and is a very complex surgery. In the UK, we have some excellent surgeons who now specialise in DIEPs, but if you're interested in this procedure, I would strongly suggest meeting with surgeons and then going with the one that you feel most confident in. Unfortunately, there can be a long waiting list for this type of surgery so if you're interested in a DIEP, this may be something you need to factor into your decision making.

Recovery from a DIEP can take some time. On average, it's around 6-12 weeks, and you'll have a very large scar that runs across your tummy (a bit like a tummy tuck, but generally, it's placed higher) and, of course, scars under your new breasts. If you've had any previous surgery on your breasts, those scars may also be visible. Whilst I don't want to liken this to a tummy tuck, it does have similar results, although the scar is typically higher than a bikini line (although there are some excellent surgeons who are known for their ability to create very low tummy scars).

Another advantage of a DIEP is that your breasts will have a very natural appearance, but they may well change shape if you put on or lose weight, so this is something to bear in mind.

The other consideration is that a DIEP may require two or three surgeries. Your tummy scar may create dog ears – little tufts of skin that stick out either side – and these may need a short surgery to correct them. In addition, you may need to have your nipples recreated (please see the section below). Tweaks may be needed to perfect the final look, so it can take a year or two to get the look you want. Of course, each surgery has downtime but nothing near to the 6-12 weeks of the initial surgery.

With a DIEP, during recovery, you will have to wear a sports-type bra, but you'll also have to wear a compression garment on your stomach. This can be challenging but is a necessity.

Latissimus Dorsi Reconstruction (LD)

The latissimus dorsi muscle is the muscle that runs either side of your back below your shoulders and is the muscle that we use for twisting and turning. This gives the LD reconstruction a unique feel in that it is typically harder than other types of reconstruction. The size of your reconstructed breasts will be dictated largely by the amount of volume or tissue that the surgeon is able to remove from your back. Occasionally, implants will be used with this reconstruction. This is a major operation because it brings muscles from the back around to the front and due to the muscle relocation, it can mean that what you're able to do in terms of movement (during exercise, for example), may be limited or painful. If you are very active and sporty, or have back or shoulder problems, this type of reconstruction is normally not suitable.

The scars from an LD reconstruction are visible on the back and also at the front, but of course, as with all surgery, the scars fade over time.

Transverse Upper Gacilis Reconstruction (TUG)

The TUG procedure is not one that is seen much now, but it can be performed if other types of surgeries have failed, or are not suitable, and can be used with or without implants.

This surgery involves using the inner thigh muscle, fat and blood vessels and relocating them to the breast area. Like the LD above, typically, only smaller breasts can be achieved with this method, although I have to say that I've seen one lady who has had the most remarkable reconstruction using this method. You can read her story, and see her photos, in the next chapter.

The scars usually run down the inside of both thighs and underneath the bottom on both sides. Of course, the breasts will also have scars, as with any mastectomy. A compression garment may have to be worn on the leg area while the areas recover.

The advantage to this surgery is that you have slimmer thighs as a result, but if only one breast is reconstructed using this method, you may want to check that both thighs will be used to avoid having different size thighs.

Other Types of Reconstruction

There are other types of reconstruction, but at the time of writing, the ones listed above are the most popular ones. There is a reconstruction that uses your own fat to create a new breast – think of having liposuction that is then put into your breast area. This does work for some ladies, but it's a long process because only a small amount can be harvested and moved at any one time. Your body can also reabsorb the harvested tissue, so it might be necessary to have the process repeated over a few years. This can be time-consuming, and the results are not guaranteed, but it can be done.

Nipple Reconstruction

With all reconstructions, you may have your nipple/areola area reconstructed. There are various options, and it really comes down to personal preference. I've listed below some of the options:

- Nipple Mounds – a small mound to represent the nipple can be recreated from your own breast tissue. The advantage of this is that it replicates a 3D affect that can be further enhanced with a tattoo to create the areola. With a DIEP, nipple mounds are typically carried out in a separate operation, but with implants, it can be done at the same time.

- Free Nipple Graft – only certain surgeons offer this option, but it's a process whereby your own nipple is reused to recreate a new nipple and areola. The surgeon will remove your existing nipples, take away as much tissue from them as possible, and then reattach in their new position. The risk is that they won't reattach and could become necrotic and die. However, this is a small risk. If your cancer was anywhere near the nipple area, this is not something that your surgeon will offer in case there are unseen cancer cells, but that's possibly the only reason why you couldn't have it. The advantages of a free nipple graft are that your nipples will always look natural and will never need further operations or upkeep. Of course, they won't have sensation as your previous nipples did, but you may find that some nerves do grow back, and they may react to temperature changes.

- 3D Tattoos – these have become incredibly popular, and the tattoos are of a medical-grade. In the hands of a great artist, you'd be hard-pressed to know they were tattoos and not natural! Either with, or without, a nipple mound, these can look amazing, and you will have a choice of colour and size. The downside, as with any tattoo, is that they can fade, and you may need top-ups to maintain colour. How often you will need this is very individual and reliant on the strength of colour used.

- Temporary Nipple Tattoos – these are as the name suggests. They can be put on in the same way as any other temporary tattoo and can last from a few days to a week. They can be purchased in lots of different colours and designs. They're not for everyone but are a good option if you want a temporary fix.

- Adhesive Nipples – these are similar to temporary tattoos, but they're applied as and when needed. These are temporary solutions but can be a morale booster.

CHAPTER 17

PATIENTS' STORIES OF SURGERY

When I was diagnosed and had to face surgical decisions, although my surgeon was fantastic at showing me different images of what a lumpectomy and mastectomy might look like, I also wanted to know what to expect. What would the scars be like? What was recovery like? Did anybody regret the surgery they'd had? It's not a decision to be taken lightly, and I felt so ill-equipped to make it.

Therefore, this chapter has real-life stories of the main types of surgery and reconstruction that are available. Please bear in mind that each surgeon has their own preferred way, so don't be surprised if something is different for you. This is purely about giving more information, showing you photographs and hopefully helping in your decision making. There is no right or wrong choice.

Lumpectomy Surgeries

Michele's Story – Lumpectomy with Sentinel Node Removal

I honestly wasn't sure what to expect from a lumpectomy and went into it only partially prepared. I think I would rather have known exactly what to expect so I knew all of it was routine and normal. At diagnosis, my scans showed I had a tumour of 9mm, and it looked like my nodes were cancer-free, so it was decided I would have surgery first.

Like most surgeries with a general anaesthetic, I wasn't allowed to eat or drink on the day, so I had got to the stage of eating a nurse by the time I was taken to the theatre! In my starving state, I was given a gorgeous gown and paper knickers, and then taken to a room with a giant scanning machine. I don't know what type of scanner it was, but it looked like half an MRI scanner - it had a bed, and then a piece of equipment would go from one side and over to the other side, but I was in the open - not closed in - so it wasn't claustrophobic like an MRI scanner.

I was first scanned for about 10 minutes - I have no idea what the purpose of that was. Then I had a colourless radioactive liquid injected into my breast! For those of you who are old enough to remember, I had visions of walking down the hospital corridor with a glow all around me, a bit like the Reddy Brek Kid!!! It was uncomfortable but bearable. I wouldn't choose to have it done every day, though! I then had to hop off the machine and walk around to encourage the liquid to move around the ducts in the breast. I also had to massage it to encourage the distribution. Ten minutes later, I hopped back onto the machine to see if the radioactive liquid had moved. Mine was being stubborn and wasn't moving, so I was told they were going to move me onto the next process before I could carry on with them.

This was the bit I was surprised about because nobody had told me that this would happen! I was taken into a room with an ultrasound machine and was told that a doctor would insert a guide wire into my breast to direct the surgeon to the right spot. Now in my head, I had assumed that this was a tiny wire that you could hardly see, and perhaps it was put in under the skin (a bit like having a marker put in at a biopsy). Errrrr, no. This was a wire that was about 40cm long! What?! OMG! I decided at this stage not to look. I'm not normally bothered by anything, but it was the thought of it more than it actually being done! The area was numbed with some gel, and all I actually felt was some tugging, pulling and pressure and then a click when it went in. The wire that was hanging out of my boob, which was probably about 30cm long, was then wound around and taped to my chest! Lovely!

The next stage was to have a mammogram to check that the wire was in the right place. Oh, for goodness sake, no! Well, yes, just get on with it, Michele! So, I had my boob squished and had to sit outside while they checked the mammogram. Guess what? "I'm so sorry, but it's in the wrong place - I'm afraid I've got to put another one in! WHAT? OMG, this can only happen to me. Okay, well, let's get on with it again! Back into the ultrasound room and push, prod, and ouch, another one goes in. I'm now looking like you can get Radio 1 if you twiddle my wires! Back for more boob squishing, and thankfully it's now in the right place (or at least the two wires cross-dissect where the surgeon needs to go). Phew! To make sure the surgeon knew which was the correct wire, the Doctor then found a pad of post-it notes and wrapped a bright pink one around the correct wire - so I now look like I'm flying a flag!

Me and my wires are sent back to the room with the big scanning machine, and I hop onto the bed. This time they confirm that the dye has indeed infiltrated all areas (I've now got the music from Mission Impossible playing in my head!), and I have to lie still for about 15 minutes while they take pictures for the surgeon to refer to during surgery. And back in the room to await being taken down to surgery!

I think I was in surgery and recovery for about 2 hours - I'm not sure because I was asleep! However, when I was back in my room, I had a quick look, and there was a bandage over both cuts (the lumpectomy and node removal scar), but I didn't feel too sore - just some mild discomfort. HOWEVER, what on earth was that just to the right of my nipple???? I've turned into a Smurf! There was a huge blue patch. I don't just mean pale blue or a hint of blue; I mean BRIGHT SMURF BLUE!

During surgery, my surgeon injected a blue dye that interacted with the radioactive dye I had put in earlier, to follow the path from the tumour to the nodes that may/may not be affected. Some five months later, I was still sporting a blue patch, but it had faded to a paler blue rather than full-on Smurf! I knew it would disappear in time, but I liked it! Another effect of the dye is that you wee the blue dye out for a few days (and weirdly, if you cry, you will cry blue tears)! If you've ever used a BlooLoo tablet in your loo, that's exactly what your wee will look like!

Even though a rather large lump had been taken out, at that point, my boob looked just the same as it had pre-surgery. I later found out that my surgeon had used some lipo-filling to fill the crater! Unfortunately, my body decided to eat it all up, and so I did have a bit of crater going on, which could have been refilled in the future if I wanted.

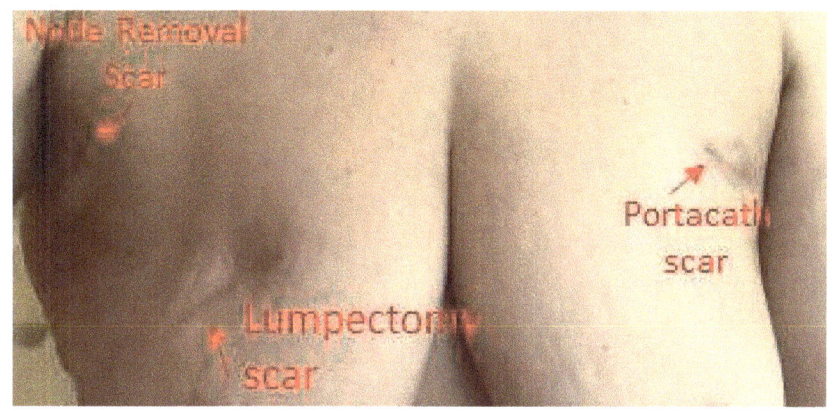

I had to wear a comfortable sports bra all day and all night for six weeks after surgery. I couldn't find a front fastening one that fitted well, was comfortable and gave me support, but in the first few weeks, it was impossible to reach behind to do up, so I had to pull the back fastening one around to the front do up, and then swivel around.

I had to go back about two weeks later for my surgery results. I forgot to mention, but I had specifically asked my surgeon to take more tissue than he thought he would normally because I wanted to make sure it was all out, and I had "clear margins". My surgeon told me he was so pleased he had done what I asked, because when the tissue was sent to the lab, not only was there a tumour (which was actually 1.5cm) but there was also a patch of DCIS that was quite large and hadn't been seen on any of my scans. Thankfully he had got it all out, with clear margins, and the lab confirmed that no cancer had been seen in the two nodes removed.

A few months after surgery, I did develop a lump under the scar where my nodes were removed. I was quite alarmed when I first found it because it was a definite lump, but it turned out to be scar tissue. The only other complication was that I developed a slight amount of cording (tightening of the muscles) down the node removal arm. When I moved my arm, it felt tight and ached a bit. I was given exercises and also had some physio on that area, and it resolved quite quickly.

Cheryl's Story – Lumpectomy with Full Node Removal

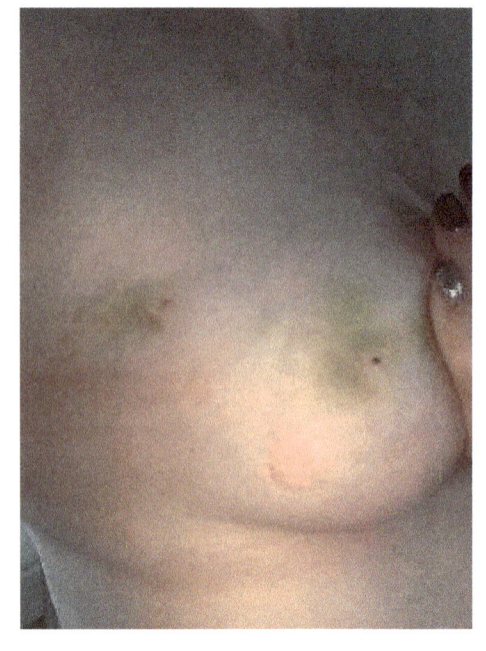

On 13th June 2020, I found a lump on the right side of my breast. I found this because it was itchy, and I had no experience or knowledge of how to check my breasts. I went to my GP 2 days later, and they referred me to the breast specialist unit. I got an appointment for 25th June (10 days after seeing my GP), and I had a mammogram, ultrasound, and biopsy. I also had a "Magseed" marker put in as well as the biopsy, and one was put in by the tumour and the other by my nodes which gave me some bruising. At that appointment, they told me that they thought it was breast cancer and was also in one of my nodes. This was such a shock, but I had to wait for the results of the biopsy.

On 7th July, I went back to the clinic, and my world came crashing down. It was confirmed that I had a 22mm Triple Negative breast cancer, but because they could see it in one node, I had to have an MRI scan, a CT scan of my abdomen and chest and a bone scan. I also had to have my blood taken to see if I had any issues with my genes.

Thankfully when I got the results of the scans, no further spread was found, but I definitely had it in my breast and in 1 node. The results of the genetic testing took longer to come back.

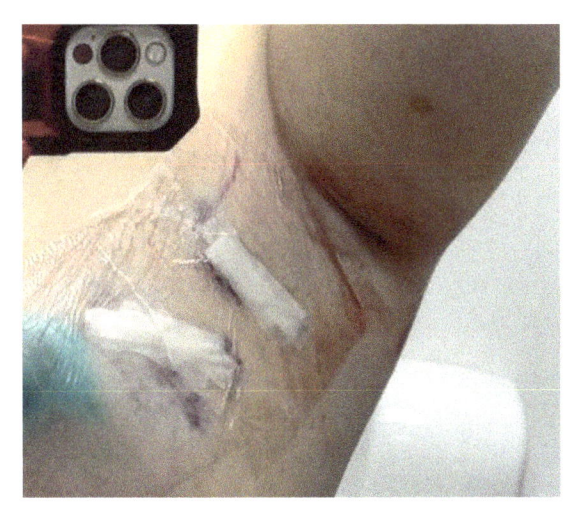

It was decided I would have chemotherapy before surgery, so I had 4 x EC and 4 x Paclitaxel with surgery afterwards. Thankfully the tumour did shrink but didn't completely disappear after chemotherapy, so it was decided

I would have surgery, radiotherapy and then Capecitabine afterwards.

Surgery was scheduled for 5th January 2021, and after surgery, I woke up with a blue patch but no drain. The surgeon removed the tumour and also three nodes, but it was then decided I would have a second surgery to clear all the nodes as a precaution.

Because of Covid and staff shortages, the second surgery didn't take place until 15th February. At that surgery, I had a drain put into the lymph node area, but it was only in overnight and taken out the next day. Unfortunately, I did have some fluid build-up after I went home, and this interfered with the healing, and I developed lymphoedema in my arm.

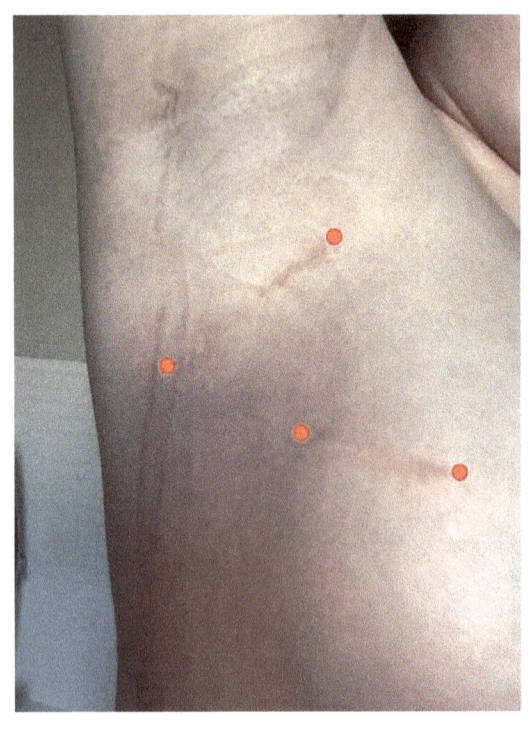

One year later, my scars have almost disappeared, but I do have to wear a compression sleeve on my arm and hand for the lymphoedema.

Natalie's Story – Lumpectomy/Node Removal Using One Scar

In November 2018, I was undressing, and as I was taking my top off, my hand brushed against my right breast, and I felt a lump. I wasn't sure if it was something new or not, but when I felt my left breast, there was nothing there. It was a weekend, so first thing on Monday morning, I rang my GP where the receptionist told me they were no appointments. When I explained that I found a lump, she said she would find a doctor to see me.

I was referred to my local breast clinic, and I had a mammogram, followed by an ultrasound. While having the ultrasound, I asked if she could see anything unusual. She did explain that cysts are usually smooth and round, but I could see my lump wasn't, and she added it was an area of concern. Then she said she would need to do a biopsy. I think that was the moment I knew it was cancer without anyone saying it. When I went to see the consultant, they said it was likely to be cancer, but they would need to confirm exactly what it was. Fast forward to 5 days before Christmas, it was confirmed as cancer, but they weren't sure what type it was.

In January 2019, it was confirmed as Triple Negative, 26mm in size. Stage 1, and grade 3. I was then given an appointment to go to St Bartholomew's Hospital in London to see Professor Schmid. He went through the treatment plan, which would be chemotherapy, surgery and then radiotherapy. However, he did ask if I wanted surgery or chemotherapy first. I opted for chemotherapy, and at this point, he also asked if I wanted to take part in an immunotherapy trial. I said yes and was chosen to have Atezolizumab.

So, I had a large dose of that first. Then three weeks later, I started 12 weekly cycles of Paclitaxel/Carboplatin with Atezolizumab every other week before the second set of chemotherapy which was 4 x fortnightly cycles of AC.

I'm a nanny, and fortunately, the children were school age, and I had very supportive bosses. They asked me what I wanted to do in terms of work, and I said I wanted to work as much as I could. So other than chemo days (Professor Schmid suggested Fridays, so I had the weekend to rest), I continued working.

I finished chemotherapy in June 2019 and had a good response to it; they couldn't pick anything up on the scans. My lumpectomy and sentinel node removal were in early August. Due to the placement of where my lump had been, they only needed to make one scar, and surgery was very straightforward, and I was home the same day. I was out and about the next day. When the dressings came off, the scar was healing nicely. The photo is two weeks after surgery.

After the surgery, however, they found 2mm of pre-cancerous cells were left, so it was suggested I have 8 cycles of Capecitabine after radiotherapy as a 'belt and braces' approach. Fortunately, I had minimal side effects, and it didn't really interfere with my day-to-day life.

After surgery, but prior to starting Capecitabine, I had 19 sessions of radiotherapy after my scar had healed and I had enough movement. I not only worked through treatment, but I also exercised, so putting my arms above my head wasn't an issue, and my radiotherapy sessions were straightforward too.

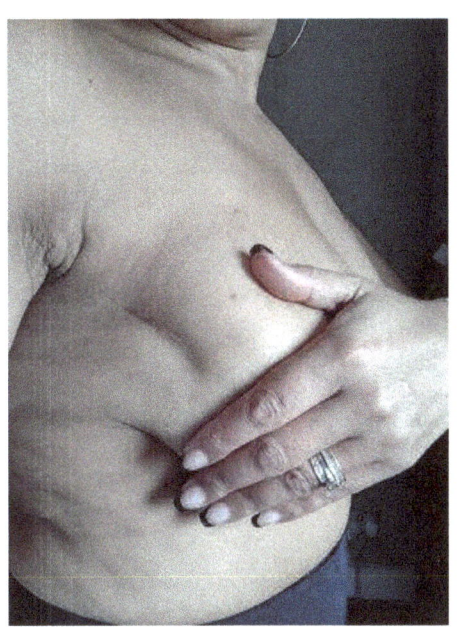

I feel very lucky that I have managed 15 months of treatment and surgery with minimal effects. One breast is smaller than the other, but other than that and my scar, which is now just over a year old, you wouldn't know unless I showed you!!

Kalie's Story – Lumpectomy - Invasive Lobular & DCIS

In 2017 I discovered cysts in my breast, so when I had pain in April 2019, I went to my GP again. She said the pain wasn't a symptom of breast cancer (something I now know is wrong), but I insisted on being checked (even though six months earlier, I'd had a mammogram that was clear).

An area of around 1.5cm showed up on the mammogram as being suspicious, but it was barely seen (which can be common with Lobular breast cancer). I couldn't feel a lump at all, and my only symptom was the pain. At the breast unit, I had a biopsy taken, and it was confirmed to be invasive breast cancer.

At surgery, it was discovered that my tumour was under a previously diagnosed cyst and was an invasive tumour of 2cm, but it was surrounded by 1cm of DCIS (normal, not lobular). I also had two nodes removed. When the laboratory report came back, it was discovered that the tumour was lobular and also had pleomorphic cells, which are more likely to spread. Also, one of the nodes removed had micromets of cancer. However, the surgeon had achieved clear margins.

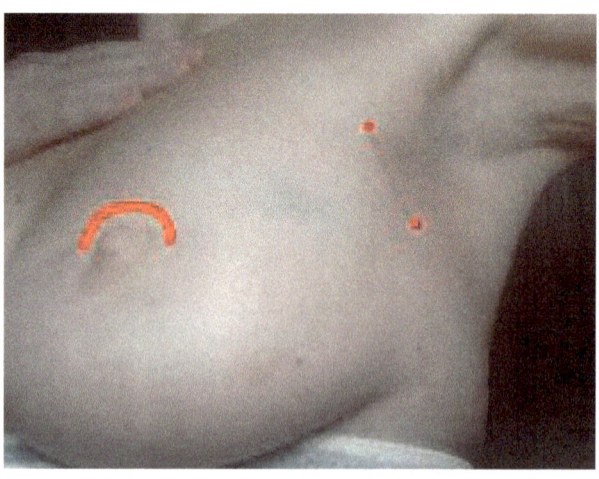

The surgeon managed to remove the tumour by cutting around my nipple from 9 o'clock to 3 o'clock as the tumour was sitting under the nipple area and just above it. This has resulted in an incredibly neat scar that can hardly be seen. The only way to tell is that the nipple is slightly upturned, and I've lost a tiny portion of the areola across the top of the nipple. I also have a scar where the nodes were removed, but this has faded and is almost invisible now. I'm very pleased with the outcome.

Chemotherapy commenced three weeks after surgery, and it was planned that I would have 3 x FEC and then 3 x Docetaxol, but unfortunately, my last Docetaxol was cancelled because I was suffering from severe peripheral neuropathy.

For me, each hospital visit was a long way from home. Chemotherapy was on the Isle of Skye, which is my nearest hospital and 3+ hours round trip by car. Since I lived alone and wasn't allowed to drive, these trips were made by the volunteer car scheme and friends. Radiotherapy was at the main hospital in Inverness (4 hours round trip), and because I had 15 sessions, I had to stay near the hospital for three weeks.

I was originally told I wouldn't get bisphosphonate treatments, but after speaking with an online group, I realised I was eligible, and when I showed my oncologist the guidelines, he agreed, and I was allowed to have them.

Nobody has ever discussed what are the implications of having a lobular invasive cancer, if any, but I've read about it, so I feel prepared if I were to ever be diagnosed again. Four months after treatment ended, I developed radiation pneumonitis, which caused breathlessness for a couple of months, and I still have peripheral neuropathy and lots of dental problems.

Melanie's Story – Lumpectomy to Mastectomy - ER+ to Triple Negative

At the beginning of December 2019, I received the dreaded news that the small lump in my left breast was a 14mm Grade 3, ER+ invasive ductal carcinoma. But the good news was that I'd only need a lumpectomy and sentinel node biopsy. It was so fantastic as it meant that by the end of January, my life would hopefully be back to normal. Unfortunately, with ER+ breast cancer (and this doesn't apply with Triple Negative), your oncologist will run an "Oncoscore", and this will determine whether you need chemotherapy or not. After all my surgeries, my oncologist told me I would, in fact, need chemo, so that was added to my treatment plan.

I did ask for a mastectomy. I just wanted the cancer gone but was told that the recurrence rates are the same, so a lumpectomy would be just as good but less invasive. I booked my operation for the week before Christmas, which for me was good timing, no school runs, and my partner always has two weeks off over Christmas, so plenty of recovery time, sitting on the sofa being waited on. I was definitely going to milk this! No pun intended!

I was relieved I could have the operation at my local hospital and not have to drive 40 minutes to the main hospital where all my breast clinic appointments had been so far, and my surgeon's name was the same as my fantastic Crohn's consultant, so I felt this was my good luck good omen.

On the morning of my operation, one of the worst things was not being able to have my morning cuppa, which always made me feel so grumpy. My partner and my then 8-year-old came onto the ward with me, and they were allowed to stay until they had to leave to do the school run. Only my family (including my two adult children) knew at this point. I didn't tell anyone else as I never wanted my 8-year-old to hear the word cancer. As far as she knew, I had a lump that was better out than in. The less she knew, the better.

I started chatting to a lady who was in the bed opposite me. I regret never getting her name as she'll never know how much she helped. She'd already had chemo and was now having her operation. She was so hopeful, so optimistic, and so full of joy that she just made me feel that everything was going to be okay.

It's amazing how quick operations go. One minute you have a cannula put in, the next you're waking up after the operation. I remember explaining to the surgeon beforehand why I had loads of scratches on my shoulders and back, as I was worried, he would think I had some sort of fetish. I have a cat that loves to jump up your back onto your shoulders, silly really, but shows how you worry about the most random things.

When I woke up, I was shocked at how painful it was, so I asked the nurse for some pain relief. She gave me one paracetamol which is all I could have apparently according to my weight! I'm pleased to say that pain relief has never been an issue with any of the operations that followed.

Before I left, the nurse read out the operation notes to me. I have no idea why she did because I didn't ask her to! What stood out was that there was an enlarged node, and she had no idea what it meant. Great! My follow up appointment was in 3 weeks, so I spent the whole-time thinking cancer had spread to my lymph nodes (which it actually hadn't). My surgeon was annoyed she had told me that.

Recovery wasn't too bad. Plenty of pillows on the bed to lie on, and I was able to drive by the time kids went back to school in January. Putting gears into reverse was a bit painful, but that was it. My ribs on the operation side felt the worst, they were so bruised and painful, and I even had bruises on my hip.

The scar on my boob was so small you couldn't really tell I'd had an operation. The line under my armpit where I'd had 3 nodes removed was bigger. It also felt really tight and burning under my arms, and I couldn't reach my arms too far above my head. I did find that bra bands hurt, so I bought a couple of zip-up mastectomy bras. They were so comfortable, so I definitely recommend them - no more underwired bras for me.

Results were back three weeks later. All the cancer had gone, but I had a patch of DCIS (pre-cancerous cells), and the surgeon felt it would be best to operate again to get out anything that had been left behind. Unbelievably, I had to have not one but two more lumpectomy operations.

The healing each time felt easier than the first lumpectomy, but I'm presuming that was because no nodes were taken again. However, I did end up having a CT scan on my ribs as so painful. To this day, they still hurt. I wasn't so much worried about the operations, but by this time, I had been told I would need chemotherapy, so I was then worried about all the knock-on treatment delays – each time, there was one week for the operation plus three weeks wait for results.

After the 3rd lumpectomy, and by now it was the end of March, the surgeon finally agreed to do a mastectomy! I only have small breasts, and they couldn't remove any more tissue without my breast having a big dent in it. I did have a choice, though, whether to have the mastectomy first or go to chemo and then have the mastectomy after. Discussing it with my surgeon, we decided on mastectomy first as covid had just hit the scene, so we were hopeful that by the time I had chemo, covid would have disappeared again. How wrong!

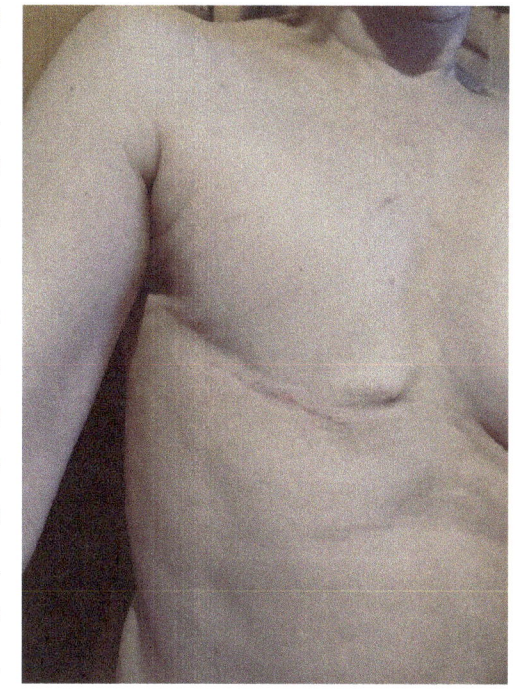

There were no options offered to have reconstruction because Covid had stopped all "non-essential" operations, but I had already decided that I didn't want one. I was tired of operations, I didn't want all the extra reconstruction ones, but above all, I was so scared of an implant hiding a recurrence. I don't even know if that is the case as the pros and cons of reconstruction have never ever been discussed with me, but as I wasn't worried about remaining flat, I didn't look into a reconstruction.

After the mastectomy, I went on to have chemotherapy and radiotherapy, and by that point, I was happy that everything was over.

Unfortunately, exactly a year later, I did have a recurrence just by my mastectomy scar. This time the tumour was Triple Negative, and I was told it was a recurrence from the previous breast cancer rather than a new primary breast cancer – although they never fully explained how they knew this.

Of course, I had to have the new cancer removed and chemotherapy again and this time radiotherapy. I now have two linear scars, but I feel the surgeon has done a marvellous job, and I'm really pleased with how it looks.

If I had a choice, I'd have a mastectomy on my other side. I have small breasts, they've been useful for breastfeeding my children, but I genuinely don't mind that I now only have one and for me, it might actually be easier having the other removed.

Mastectomy Surgeries with Reconstruction

Michele's Story – Double Mastectomy - Immediate Implants

Let's be honest.... my boobs were not attractive. Losing weight, having a child and then, more importantly, having cancer, not to mention being 54 years old, had taken a toll on them, and they weren't a pretty sight! Couple that with the fact that they had tried to kill me. It would seem like a "no brainer" to have a mastectomy. HOWEVER, it's not quite as easy as that. With a mastectomy, your nipples lose all feeling, and you may feel okay about this, but it's a big consideration. Also, if you want a reconstruction, your surgeon is unlikely to say "you'll be a C cup" - they will give you what they can, with what they have to work with, so having an implant reconstruction (like other reconstructions) can be an unknown.

I researched and agreed with my surgeon that I would have pear-shaped implants (as opposed to round), silicone and ones that had a high profile, i.e., would give more of an outward projection of a natural breast. With implant breast reconstruction, getting a good profile is more challenging than in a cosmetic boob job because there is less skin to work with. In 2017, my surgeon used Mentor High Profile silicone implants, and these were the ones during my research, which appeared to give a very good result. My surgeon also discussed the pros and cons of placing the implant above or below the muscle. I had both options, but with his guidance,

I chose under the muscle as I was worried that I had quite thin skin and the implant might be more noticeable if it was on top of the muscle.

I had set my heart on having 3D nipples tattooed after surgery, but my surgeon suggested I have a free nipple graft. This is when your own nipples are removed, the skin thinned and then reattached to the newly constructed breasts. This can't be done in all cases, and not all surgeons offer it, but after some consideration (i.e., they would look natural, and I wouldn't have to have the tattoos re-done every few years), I decided to go ahead. All these decisions are individual and need to be discussed with your surgeon because what's right for me may not be for you.

Once all the decisions were made, it was on to surgery. I had expected to feel very anxious the nearer I got, and I found every so often I questioned whether I was doing the right thing, but I kept reminding myself why it was important. So, the only real day of panic was the actual day of the operation.

I arrived at the hospital at 7 am and knew that I was going to be first down to surgery. For some reason, I had got it in my head that it was a 2-hour operation - I have no idea where I got that from, so I was floored when the anaesthetist told me I'd be sedated for around 6-8 hours! He also said I would wake up in recovery and would spend the first night in Intensive Care, followed by a second night on the ward. This was precautionary as I have diabetes, and so extra care was taken to monitor my insulin/blood sugar levels.

My surgeon came in next to draw on me, so he had a record of placement etc., and it made me realise just how much I was in his hands. I've always had faith in him. He's always given me the worst-case scenario (expect the worst and hope for the best), but I secretly knew that he would do his best. I knew he listened when I banged on relentlessly about needing perky boobs and having symmetry, and he nodded politely when I showed him inspirational photos! How he didn't ask the anaesthetist to knock me out then and there, I don't know!

Then it was time to put on the gown and paper knickers. Honestly, who designed those things? They're like giant see-through nappies! Really, really, not a good look and then it was a walk down to theatre.

I woke up in recovery at about 2.30-3.00 pm and was told everything had gone well and I had been in the theatre for just over 6 hours. Of course, the first thing I did was look down! The nipple areas were covered by sponge dressings, and I had large white bandages under each breast and steri-strips going up from under the breast to the nipple, BUT they looked amazing. Natural, and like real breasts! Not only was I happy, but the two nurses looking after me stepped back, and both said "wow"! They see a fair number of reconstructions but not many by my surgeon. They were incredibly impressed - as was I.

By this point, all I felt was overwhelming relief, the happiness it was over, and a sense of total calm. I wondered if I'd have regrets, but I had none. In fact, it was the opposite. I was thrilled - not something I had expected at all.

It was also at this point I realised I had drains in! I had one on each side (I believe some people have two on each side). There's a thin tube that goes into your body, and then about a metre down, it's linked to a wider tube that leads down to a vacuum construction at the end.

I was given two shoulder bags (one for each side), and they became my companions for the next seven days. I was shown how to empty the drains and record how much fluid came out each day. For me, the drains were the worst bit. I felt totally stuck to a chair and when I walked about was conscious of them - it was horrible - especially as our new kitten thought they were a new toy for him! Having said that, most people don't have any issue with them, so I was just being soft!

Before I was allowed home, I was visited by the hospital physio, who gave me a chart of exercises to do. To be honest, the ones you can do with drains in, I found so easy as I had quite a bit of mobility. When the drains came out, it was another story - the exercises are designed to stretch everything, and oh boy, did I feel it. On the first day of doing those, I lay on the floor, trying to get my arms above my head. It was so painful, and I got stuck and then couldn't get up. Luckily hubby was at home, and between us, we managed to get me on the sofa! Not being able to pull somebody up with their arms or under their arms is problematic!

On release from the hospital, I was given pain medication, but I found that by day 4, I didn't need anything apart from the occasional painkiller at night because when you stay still without moving, things can stiffen up a bit. The only time that my breasts hurt was when I bent forward as I got a shooting pain. So, I quickly learned not to do that!

Sleeping sitting up was problematic and uncomfortable, but it's necessary to allow the drains to work, so I bought some V-shaped pillows (like the ones you have during pregnancy) and put two behind me (normal pillows kept slipping down), and then I put normal pillows on either side of me to stop me rolling sideways. By day six, my breasts were settling down, and there was definitely less swelling.

My surgeon had left me with strict instructions that NOBODY should touch the dressings until I saw him in a fortnight. For the nipple graft to work, they have to have time to grab onto the underlying skin and attach to a blood supply, so they had to stay in place.

On day 7, I had my drains out. A painless process and best if you relax. The stitch (holding them in) is cut on either side, and then the nurse, while you take a deep breath in, literally pulls the tube out. It feels so strange coming out - not painful - but the thought of it is worse than it actually is. Within a minute, both drains were out, and a small steri-strip dressing was put over them.

Despite the swelling going down, I was still very swollen at this stage, and all the post-mastectomy bras I had bought didn't fit me. So, after having my drains out, I went straight to the bra shop and exchanged them for ones that fit.

On day 14, I saw my surgeon for the great unveiling, removal of dressings and lab results from the tissue removed at the mastectomy.

As the bandages came off, I looked down, and the nipple on my non-cancer boob I recognised immediately as my own! I didn't expect that. The right one was 75%, okay, but there was an issue in one area, and it was looking a bit black. You could still see it was my nipple, and the shape was there, and honestly, unless you knew, I don't think you'd realise that anything wasn't 100% right, but it looked more oval than the other.

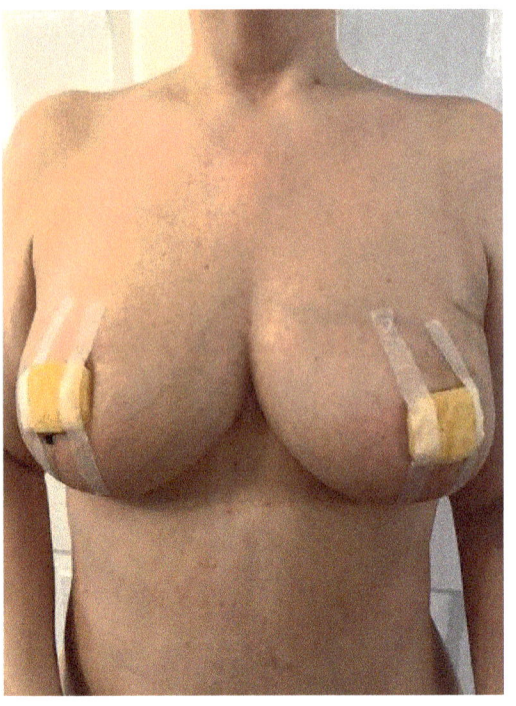

The icing on the cake? Results from the laboratory confirmed that none of the breast tissue showed any signs of cancer.

So here is the result at eight weeks post-surgery! At about 5-6 weeks, I was allowed to take the covers off the nipples. The one nipple that we thought might suffer from some necrosis hadn't and was the same colour all over but a slightly different shape to the other, possibly from being squashed by the bras. This hasn't bothered me over the years, so I've left well alone.

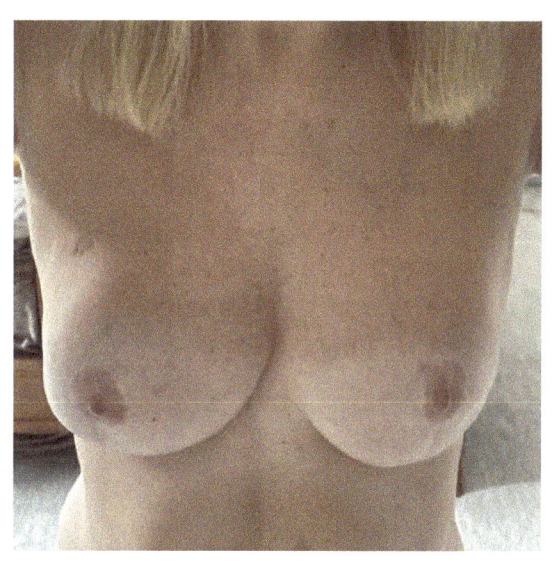

And six years later? I'm still thrilled, and it occurred to me that my breasts are the youngest thing about my body! They don't look bad on a 58-year-old! Regrets? None at all. I'm delighted beyond words. I do mourn the loss of feeling, BUT they look so much better than my old boobs and (hopefully) they won't try to kill me again! I won't downplay that this was an enormous decision to make, but I haven't for one minute regretted it. It was so important to me to do this, and I'm very, very, very pleased with the result.

Vicki's Story – Double Mastectomy - Immediate DIEP

This is my story of a double mastectomy with immediate DIEP reconstruction …. essentially using my chocolate-cake belly to make my new boobs.

My story started in 2018 when a routine yearly mammogram (although I was under 50 years old, I was being screened yearly due to a family history of ovarian and breast cancers), where they found what turned out to be a 1cm grade 3 Triple Negative breast cancer. As it was small, the decision was made to go for a lumpectomy first, then chemotherapy whilst the genetic testing was carried out. My lovely breast surgeon, being aware of the potential need for a mastectomy should a faulty gene be found, planned ahead, making sure that the lumpectomy scar would be hidden in the fold of my breast.

Well, I had a feeling that I would be the next Angelina Jolie, as lo and behold, they found I had a faulty BRCA1 gene. My breast surgeon explained that there would be a 50% chance of getting another breast cancer further down the line, but I didn't need to be convinced. I wanted a double mastectomy. I put all thoughts of that on hold, though, as the most important thing was to have chemotherapy.

As I approached my last few cycles of chemotherapy, I saw my breast surgeon again. She explained that if I would like, she could perform a double mastectomy with immediate implants (she pulled some implants out of her drawer and showed me pictures of her work), but if I wanted to go for a DIEP, she would need to refer me to a plastic surgeon at a hospital further away. What really surprised me was that she would then travel to the other hospital to perform the mastectomy alongside the plastic surgeon.

Anyway, I left that meeting carrying a bundle of leaflets so that I could have a think about what I wanted to do. The recovery time for the DIEP is much longer, but Implants may need further operations, so I was going back and forth thinking about the pros and cons. What seemed to tip the balance in my decision making were a number of ladies in a Facebook DIEP group saying that implants sometimes feel really cold, almost as if they are not part of you. However, DIEP reconstruction uses your own tissue (in my case, chocolate belly), so it is warm. I considered myself as being pretty robust, and I was talented in cultivating my belly (for the sake of my reconstruction, of course)!!

So, I met with my breast surgeon and let her know my decision. She recommended a surgeon in East Grinstead, and she sent off the referral letter. Pretty quickly, I was phoned by the hospital and offered an appointment. He talked me through everything highlighting all the risks and explaining that the operation itself would take about 9 hours and that I would wake up in a high dependency area of the ward, to be monitored frequently through the night. He explained that they would need to check the veins in my belly to see if they would be usable to replumb into my chest area. This would involve a CT scan.

Once I finished chemotherapy in spring 2019, planning for my operation kicked into gear. I was given a June date and went along to have my CT scan. I still had my PICC line in, and as they needed a line for the dye, I suggested they use it (as my veins were, and still are, really tiny and hard to find). This was a big mistake!! I learned, and so did the CT scan staff that PICC lines are not suited to the pressure used by the machine that injects the dye. The connector attached to the PICC line pinged across the room mid scan, and the dye went everywhere, me, the floor, the scanner. Anyway, after much scurrying around, they found their best vein finder and the scan was done. Tummy veins were found to be good.

The operation day approached. As I lived a distance away from the hospital, they admitted me the day before. I was given awful energy drinks to drink in the evening before and morning of the operation. I then tried to sleep - in my head saying goodbye to potential killer boobies.

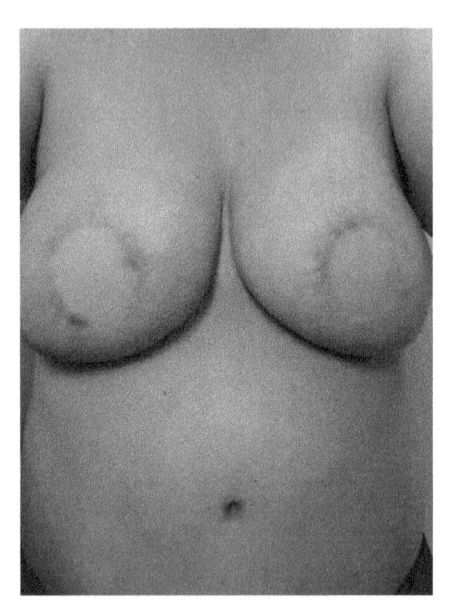

So, the morning arrived. I had a shower, put on my hospital gown, gorgeous paper knickers and sexy surgery stockings and sat waiting in my chair to be collected. Then suddenly I was off, walking with a lovely nurse trying to distract me by talking rubbish. I was put into a curtained area, and a nurse gave me a foil backed blanket, which she said was needed to keep my boob area warm (I guess to get the veins all ready for the operation).

I was then visited by the plastic surgeon and his junior, who took a very long time drawing over my tummy and boobs. At this point, my breast surgeon arrived and peeked her head around the curtain. The small curtained off area was full! Then off they went saying "See you in there"! I was walked to a bed, the anaesthetist got cracking and off I went to sleep.

I was told that I would be given a button to self-administer painkillers when I awoke from surgery. However, when I woke up, I thought I was making noises indicating that I needed all of it immediately, so I was dosed up to the eyeballs. I was wheeled round to intensive care (due to staffing issues, this was deemed the best place), and I lay there spaced out and so tired while I had oxygen, a catheter, inflatable leg things and a heated blanket on. Regularly, the nurses came round to use a doppler on my new boobs to check that blood was still flowing. This carried on all through the night.

The following morning, the catheter was removed, and a nurse gave me a bed bath!!! (Oh my word, I felt like a fragile old lady). I had a post-surgery bra put on, and I wore normal knickers, then over the top, a big pair of almost up to my armpits granny support knickers. All the while, I was being very careful of the three drains, one for each boob and one for the tummy. I felt like Neo in the matrix with all these tubes/lines coming out of me.

A nurse started mentioning getting out of bed!!!! Anyway, I don't know how I did it, but with one nurse on each side, I carefully managed to manoeuvre into a chair. Next, a physiotherapist arrived. I was given a frame to lean on (I certainly felt like an old lady), and I gradually walked slowly across the room (a snail could have lapped me), then slowly back to the chair. I seemed to have passed the physiotherapist's tests as that was the last I saw of him.

The next challenge was going to the bathroom. A nurse helped me across the room and waited while I took the longest time trying to wrestle the granny pants that felt like they were made of concrete down whilst gingerly negotiating past the tummy drain line!!! Anyway, I did it and made it back to my bed for a well-earned rest. Next, I was transferred out of intensive care to the normal ward. Gradually hour by hour, day by day, I started to get more mobile and able to shower.

My surgeon is a fan of tape to cover all scars on the breast and tummy area. So, after showering, this tape needed to be dried thoroughly using a hairdryer. I had a skin (but not nipple) sparing mastectomy, so I had breast mounds that were completely smooth which was a bit weird to start off with. There was a plan to have nipples created and then coloured in using tattooing further down the line.

I spent three nights in hospital before my drains were removed and I was allowed home. I could walk short distances but stooped over like a little old lady (giving me really bad backache), but I couldn't walk around the hospital to the car, so my husband (at the time, another story) and my son wheeled me out of the hospital and into the car for the journey home. TOP TIP, slip-on shoes, baggy trousers (not jeans), and button-up loose tops are the way to go here. And if you have any of the heart-shaped pillows you can buy, make use of them. They are fab for cushioning your new boobs from the seatbelt on the way home.

So, I got home and set up camp on the sofa with a large V-shaped pillow, duvet, remote control etc. I decided that I would sleep on the sofa, propped up in my little nest using the V-pillow and a wedge pillow for under my knees (so as not to strain tummy scar). I gradually started to recover day by day, starting out walking a short distance in the garden and then for longer and longer distances each day. I eventually started to straighten up, which helped with the backaches.

Anyway, time went by. I healed up nicely (with a few minor issues requiring the use of non-adhering dressings), and I was very impressed with both the size and shape of my breasts and the flat tummy with the lowest tummy scar that I had ever seen!

I was due to have the next phase, to lift both sides a little, to even up my right side a little, and to create nipples (using the skin and twisting it into shape), but then the pandemic hit! However, I put myself on the short notice list, and in September 2020, I was lucky enough to have this operation. It was done under general anaesthetic, so I had to stay overnight, and I woke with little cushions with holes cut out where my new nipples were happily shielded!

In 2021 my local breast surgeon tattooed my fake nipples and areolas, and honestly, I think they are much better than my originals!! I am so happy. All I need now is to find someone (other than my breast surgeons) to appreciate them. My divorce was finalised last year, and if I ever meet someone in the future, I have no concerns as far as my fantastic new boobs are concerned. What a lucky man he would be is all I can say!!

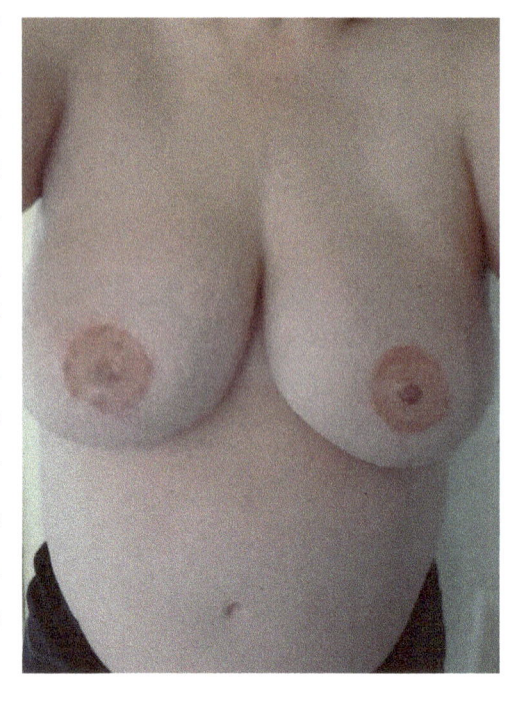

Di's Story – Double Mastectomy - Immediate DIEP

This is the story of my DIEP reconstruction... A DIEP flap is a type of breast reconstruction in which blood vessels called deep inferior epigastric perforators (DIEP), as well as the skin and fat connected to them, are removed from the lower abdomen, and transferred to the chest to reconstruct a breast after mastectomy without the sacrifice of any of the abdominal muscles.

First of all, I went to see one of the Plastic Surgery nurses who specialise in breast reconstruction. She went through all the various types of reconstruction available and showed me images of each, with before and after pictures. Up until this point, I had been very chatty and happy, as it is comforting for any woman having a mastectomy to know they will have a new breast made or breasts if having a bilateral mastectomy, which I was. The remaining flat was not an option I was willing to consider for me personally. Seeing the images (some were quite brutal) made me actually realise what I was going to go through, and yes, it was upsetting. This wasn't a cosmetic boob job, but it was the best I was going to get, and that was good enough! I would advise having your partner or a friend with you at this appointment as it can be quite emotional for some.

Due to the complexity of the surgery, few breast centres offer DIEP flap breast reconstruction. The operating time may be twice as long as with the muscle-sparing free TRAM, and the blood flow to the DIEP flap may not be as good as that of the muscle-sparing TRAM operation—something to seriously consider prior to choosing this method.

I already had a good idea that the DIEP procedure was what I was going to choose (I knew my hospital offered this type of recon) but needed that reassurance going through the other options. Implants were not an option for me as I was going to require radiotherapy following surgery. I was told from the beginning that implants would be damaged by the radiation; therefore, they would not consider offering me this type of reconstruction. Some other procedures gave a smaller sized result. DIEP felt right for me as it would give me good-sized breasts and also a tummy tuck at the same time. I was a good candidate for this surgery as I had enough of a tummy to make two new breasts, a tummy that would soon become flatter than I could ever imagine. I had a second planning appointment, this time with the plastic surgeon himself, who confirmed I was able to have this procedure. I was told not to lose any weight before surgery as he just had enough to work with. Every cloud...

A CT scan was required for preoperative imaging of the blood vessels in the abdomen. This, too, will be part of the requirements of your surgeon to confirm eligibility for this technique. They may be able to use a previous CT scan or may require another one with contrast.

As I was having a bilateral mastectomy and immediate DIEP reconstruction, I was pretty anxious about the length of time I would be in theatre. I was told it would take 10-12 hours, but in reality, I was in the theatre for 14 hours. Obviously, if you are only having one breast removed and reconstructed, this will take less time, or perhaps your reconstruction will be delayed with you already having undergone your mastectomy surgery separately. Your surgeon will advise how long the procedure is likely to take in your case.

I went into the hospital the day before surgery for the usual preoperative checks and also to be marked for surgery. Earlier in the day, I was really anxious and tearful at times, but in the evening, I managed to calm down and focus on the fact that the operation would remove the cancer, which is, of course, the most important part. I slept okay, and when I woke up on the day of surgery, everything happened in a whirlwind, and I was shortly being wheeled down to theatre. I bubbled and sobbed the whole way down. Before I knew it, I was waking up in recovery.

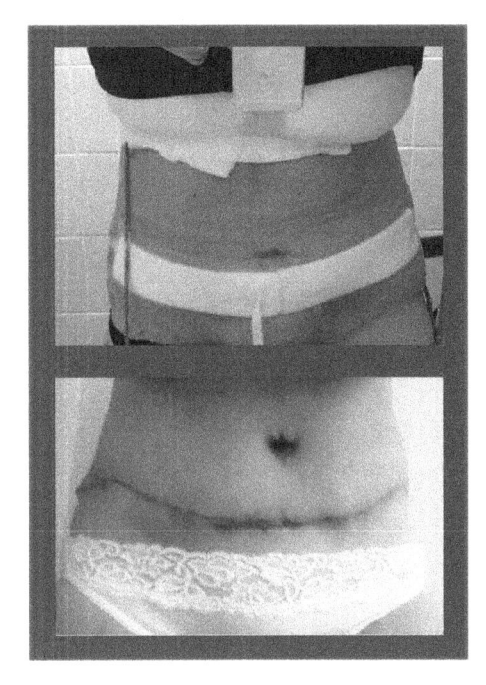

Please be prepared for possible back and shoulder pain due to being on the operating table for such a long period of time. For me, this was the worst pain in the hours that followed soon after surgery. My nurses quickly established pain relief to get this under control. When in recovery and back in the ward, I was under 30-minute observations by a nurse who was with me all night, and this continued to the first day. They need to check all the usual observations, but additionally, they need to ensure the new breast(s) has good blood flow, and there are no signs of failure. If any serious complications arose, my surgeon warned me that I might be taken back into theatre. The nurses' observations decreased to hourly, two hourly and so on as I continued to recover. It is vital that the breasts are kept warm to keep the blood flow.

Day 1 was a tough day. The simplest of tasks, like a bed bath, was quite painful as moving even a fraction hurt. I had four drains. My stomach was cut from hip to hip, but my chest, strangely, was the least painful in the early days. My four drains were one on either side of my hip and one on the outside of each breast. The drains didn't cause pain but were a pest as they got in the way. When buying nightwear or daywear for hospitals, consider low cut hipster style bottoms as the drains catch on your PJ trousers, leggings etc.

Day 2, I managed to get out of bed, and I was encouraged to do this, and it's worth the effort, trust me. Even if it's just to visit the bathroom, I was not able to stand up entirely straight, so don't be alarmed if you cannot straighten for the first few weeks. Each day I managed to do something little more than I could do the day before, but the recovery was very slow. I was in the hospital for seven days, then off home to begin my recovery alone.

Once I was on my feet, the nurses gave me drain bags that look like something you'd make in sewing at school. That meant I could pop the bags over my shoulders when walking. They are keen to remove the drains as quickly as possible to avoid infection. My consultant decided when they could be removed based on how much fluid/blood was still draining.

Showering was very difficult, and I needed help in the first few days because the dressings needed to be waterproofed, and with drains to contend with, an extra pair of hands was needed.

To assist with managing pain, I made sure I kept on top of my painkillers, trying never to miss a dose. I wore a soft, supportive bra (not wired) at all times, and took the strain off of my stomach with a pillow under my knees.

The first moment I stood in front of a mirror, alone, taking in my new body, I was pleasantly surprised. My surgeons had done a remarkable job, and my new breasts were full, natural, and perky! This, along with my incredibly flat stomach, was such a relief to see. I cried with relief - it was much better than I expected. Just be prepared for a pretty brutal looking scar to your tummy, which will, of course, fade over time and of course, you no longer have nipples (unless you are eligible for nipple-sparing surgery).

Sleeping was pretty uncomfortable at home as you no longer have the hospital bed to move into the exact position of comfort. I was advised to sleep upright and to wear a soft bra for many weeks, all day, and all night, to ensure I had full support as my new breasts settled.

My advice would be that it's really important to look after yourself and your scars and not to attempt to do anything more than your body will allow. Listen to your body. If you can, ask friends and family to help with laundry and housework for the first few weeks. If you live alone, perhaps arrange to stay with someone when you first come out of the hospital. Let people look after you.

I continued to visit my clinic weekly as healing continued and to have the dressings changed until they were happy to dismiss me. I did have complications and required an additional couple of operations in the first six weeks. This was due to some skin/tissue dying. Necrosis is very common after breast surgery, and I had a patch of necrosis that meant I needed further surgery to remove it. I was warned that I might feel lumps soon after as well and not be alarmed.

At nine weeks post-surgery, I was recovering well and returned to work a few weeks later. I needed several more operations for cosmetic improvements once things settled down as I had one breast smaller than the other due to the additional operations where they had to remove dead skin and tissue. I wasn't concerned about that, nor was my surgeon (who restored the shape he had initially after my original surgery).

If I had to do this all again, I wouldn't change a thing. It hasn't been easy, but it was the right surgery for me and worth the difficult days to see the end result.

Carley's Story – Double Mastectomy - Immediate TUG

On 20th December 2015, I found a lump in my left breast. The following day I went to the doctor. I was 34 years old at the time. My doctor referred me to a hospital, and two weeks later, I had my appointment. As you can imagine, I spent Christmas and New Year worrying.

At the appointment, I was examined by a doctor and given an ultrasound scan and had 2 biopsies taken and was told it looked clinically benign, and the next time they see me, I would hopefully be given the all-clear! I wasn't given a mammogram as they told me that I was too young. A letter that the hospital wrote to my doctor said, "Ultrasound showed 1.5cm hypoechoic oval lesion with a slightly lobulated border and is likely to represent a fibroadenoma" and confirmed that core biopsies were taken.

I had an appointment for two weeks later on a day that I was supposed to be at work, so I asked if they could change it to a few days later as in my head, I was going to be okay! On the day of my appointment, I told my husband to go to work, but my friend insisted she come with me, so I wasn't on my own. When we got to the hospital, I told my friend I was okay, and she could wait in the waiting room, and I walked into the room. The doctor said, "have you anyone with you?" and that's when I knew it was bad news. I burst into tears, and they told me I had cancer, and the Macmillan nurse got my friend. I didn't take anything in at that point, and my friend rang my husband, who came home.

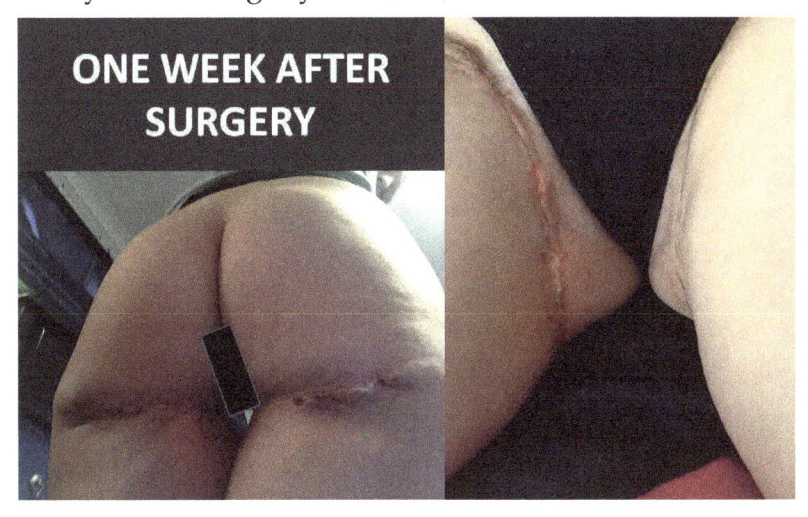

ONE WEEK AFTER SURGERY

The next day I had a mammogram, another biopsy, but this time from my lymph nodes and a CAT scan. When the results came back, it confirmed that I had "left breast intraductal carcinoma 1.5cm in diameter, grade 3, Triple Negative, lymph node-positive". I then had to have an MRI and also a bone scan, but thankfully those were both clear.

However, because of my age, it was decided that I should have genetic testing, even though there was no family history. The Doctors wanted to get the results from the testing back before surgery, so the decision was that I should have chemotherapy first. I have a real fear of needles, so I had a portacath inserted the day before my first chemo. My chemo regime was 3 x FEC and 3 x Docetaxel with a Zoladex injection every month to protect my ovaries whilst on chemo. Halfway through chemo, I was given another ultrasound that showed the lump had shrunk by a third and had responded really well.

The genetic results came back and confirmed I was BRCA2 positive. At that point, I decided I wanted to have a double mastectomy and so started to investigate reconstruction options. I didn't have enough fat on my tummy for a DIEP and also didn't want implants, so my surgeon suggested I have the TUG procedure (where fat/skin is taken from the inner thigh).

On 21st June 2016, I had my operation (which included full node clearance on my left-hand side – the side that had breast cancer). The operation was about 10 hours, and all the cancer was removed with good margins (so my surgeon later told me that I wouldn't need radiotherapy). During recovery, I was put under a heating blanket to keep the new breast tissue warm. I also had two drains in each breast to drain away from the excess fluid and one drain to each thigh (which were the last ones to come out).

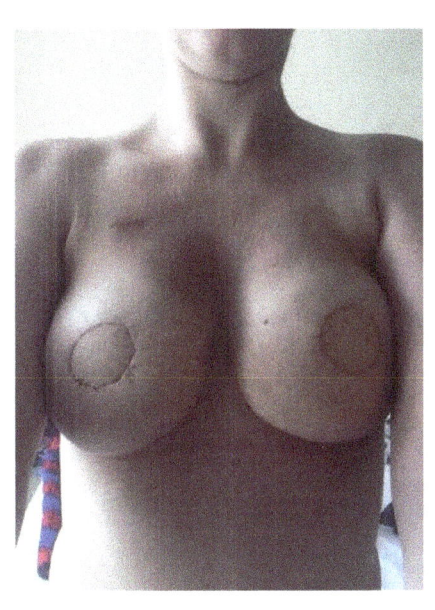

I was in the hospital for 6 days, and the pain in the thigh area was definitely more painful than the breast area. The cut on the thigh extends around and under my bottom at the back and then up into the inner groin area, so it was extensive, and the photo was taken a week after surgery. However, I was only home for two days when they split open, and I got an infection. I was re-admitted for four days and put on intravenous antibiotics. My thighs were horrendous, and I had to have my dressings changed every other day due to them leaking excess fluid. They definitely took much longer to heal than my breasts. My thighs took about 3 or 4 months to fully heal.

By contrast, the photo on the next page of my breasts was taken six weeks after the operation, and they healed beautifully. They felt very natural and soft, and exactly like my breasts felt before surgery, and I'm thrilled with them. I decided not to have nipple reconstruction as I didn't want any tissue to remain from my breasts. In the photo on the previous page, you'll see that there are circles where my nipples would be. During the operation, the skin covering the breasts is saved, and the tissue from the thighs is put under to make the breast. However, the surgeons need a way to check how the tissue under the breast is responding, and therefore a small area is left that exposes the thigh tissue underneath. Any changes in colour etc., may indicate a problem, but I didn't have any of that. They also checked the tissue was okay by using a Doppler every 15 minutes for the first 24hrs, then every 30 minutes and then every hour etc., so there was lots of checking!

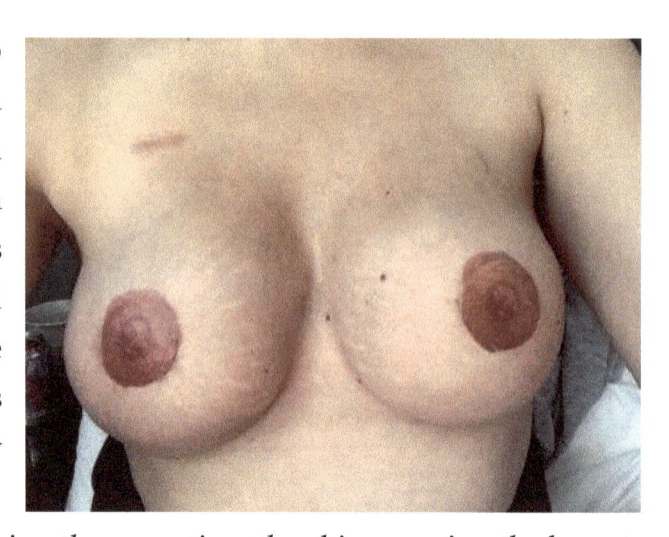

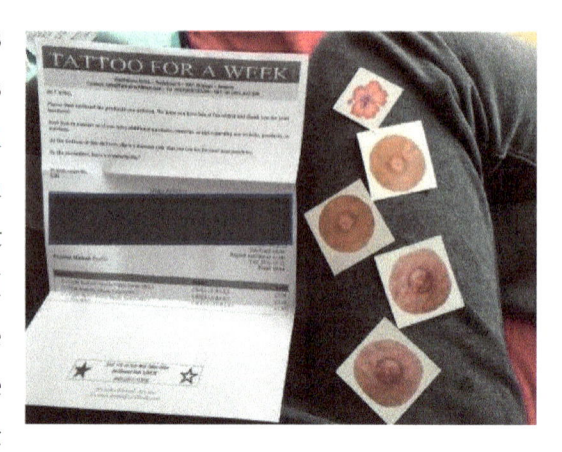

Where the circles are on the breast is where tattoos will create the nipple area once fully healed, but in the meantime, I found some temporary nipple tattoos that you put on, and they last for about a week before you need to replace them. It's an American store but offers lots of different sizes and colours.

At 15 weeks post-surgery, I was still wearing a soft bra, day, and night, and I will have had (at some point) a bilateral oophorectomy (i.e., taking my ovaries out) as with BRCA2 there is an increased risk of ovarian cancer, but we've delayed this as we would like to try for another baby.

I am delighted with my reconstruction option, but, like all reconstructions, it was tough going but worth it in the long run.

Kath's Story – Double Mastectomy - Immediate LD

Well, this is my journey, and I hope it helps somebody who's looking for some information about the LD (Latissimus Dorsi) reconstruction.

In November 2009, I was diagnosed with breast cancer in my right breast. The cancer was Grade 3 and HER2+. I was told that I could have a lumpectomy which I was very relieved about, and I had the lumpectomy first followed by chemotherapy radiotherapy, and then because it was HER2+, I had 18 treatments of Herceptin. So, all in all, my treatment lasted a little over 18 months. In November 2011, I had a mammogram, and that was all clear. I was then discharged by the Oncology Team and referred to the Breast Unit to have regular check-ups.

My first appointment with the Breast Unit was in May 2012, and they found a lump in my left breast. This time, it was Grade 3 (the same as before), but it was Triple Negative and not HER2+. I was referred back to Oncology, and they gave me the choice of a lumpectomy or mastectomy to that breast. I decided to have a single mastectomy because I really didn't want to go through everything again. We discussed all reconstruction options, but I didn't have enough fat on my tummy area for the DIEP reconstruction, and I was told that although I could have implants, there was less chance of rejection, and my breast would have a more natural feel/look if I had the LD reconstruction and nipple reconstruction at the same time (using the skin from my back as well). I have never been offered tattooed nipples, but I'm quite happy with my reconstructed ones, so that's not a problem for me.

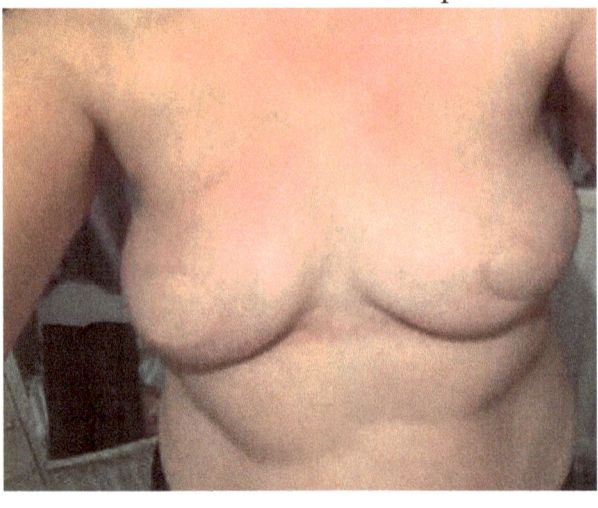

The operation took 6 hours, and when I woke up, I was in pain for a few days, but this did get better. For the first day or two, it's really important to keep the breast area warm (to aid the blood supply), so the nurses put a special heat blanket on me. I also had three drains in the breast that were draining the fluid away and the fluid reduced significantly over the next five days. I was discharged from the hospital after 5 days and went home. I had to wear a soft bra for 6 weeks (all day and all night) to help with the healing process, and I wasn't too uncomfortable, but sleeping was a bit difficult, so my husband temporarily moved into the spare room. Some ladies find a V-shaped pillow helpful for support (the type used during pregnancy).

In January 2015, I made the decision to go back and have a mastectomy on my right side (the side that had HER2+ cancer). I made this decision because I wanted to be in control before any new cancer made the decision for me.

This operation took a little longer than the first mastectomy and was 7 hours, but I recovered very well afterwards. I was given an injection in my back during the operation, which really with the pain management.

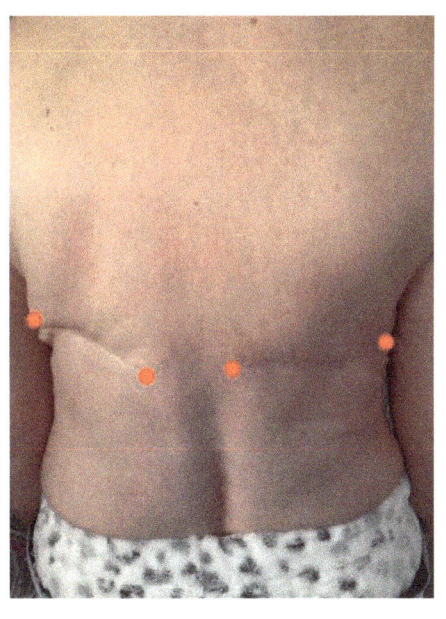

Both scars on my back are covered by my bra (not everybody's scar will be hidden by their bra because of their anatomy as it can be above or below the bra line). As this procedure uses the muscle from the back, it's fairly common that patients can have some restriction or pain in the back area as an ongoing issue. I do get uncomfortable sometimes in my back area, but I have absolutely no regrets and am now over 10 years clear.

Mastectomy Surgeries with No Reconstruction

Sheila's Story – Single Mastectomy with No Reconstruction

In January 2016, I cricked a muscle in my neck and went to see the GP. She spotted I hadn't been called to attend a mammogram the year before when I turned 50, so she arranged for me to have one. At my first routine mammogram, there was an incidental finding of shadowing but no lumps. I re-attended the clinic a week later for a core biopsy on the shadow area, which showed an invasive ductal carcinoma with negative receptors to ER, PR, and HER.

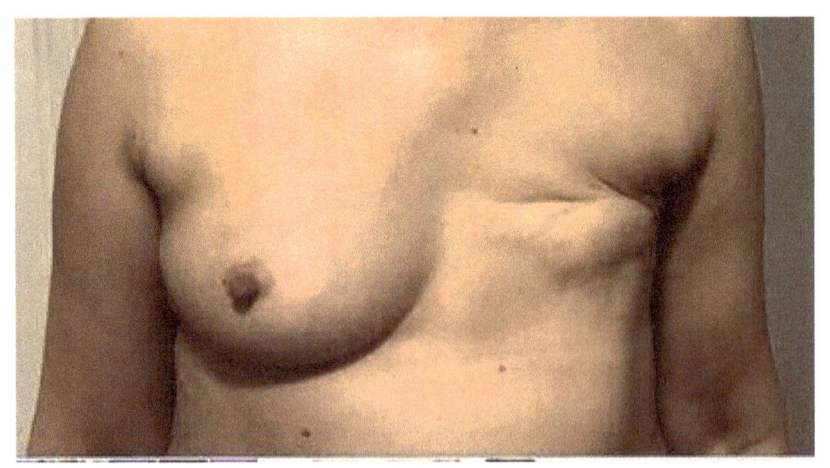

As I had very small breasts, the surgeon didn't offer a lumpectomy as he explained it would be too difficult to make sure he had taken the tumour out and also surrounding tissue to get clear margins, leaving enough breast tissue to form a breast. Also, my tumour was against my chest wall at the back, so reconstruction wasn't offered at that point. So, three weeks later, I had a left mastectomy and sentinel node biopsy. The results came back with the official diagnosis of a 22mm grade 2 Invasive Ductal Carcinoma along with a high-grade Ductal Carcinoma In-situ of 10mm as well as lymphovascular invasion. Only one out of the four nodes removed was positive, and I had clear margins.

On the morning of the surgery, I just wanted this 'thing' gone, so I was anxious but not overly upset. As I am quite small-breasted, the whole breast had to be removed to ensure a clear margin around the tumour site. When I awoke, I felt surprisingly felt calm. I had a drain leading from the surgery site, and overnight very little leaked into the drain, so I was discharged with a 'softie' and post-mastectomy bra.

As chemotherapy and radiotherapy followed over the next 6-7 months, I didn't really have time to think about the loss of a breast. Treatments were so aggressive (FEC-T x 6 cycles 3 weeks apart and 15 radiotherapy blasts over 15 days to the chest wall and axilla), and I had to be hospitalised three times.

Once it was over, I focused on LIVING again; my children were 19,15 and 11. The eldest had gone to university, and the baby had started senior school. I was devastated that I had not been able to have that summer with them.

In May 2017, I had a review with the plastic surgeon and was offered a reconstruction with a tummy tuck (DIEP). Before the date of the operation, I made the decision NOT to have reconstruction. It dawned on me that I was now healthy, happy at a second chance at life, my boobs had done their 'job' when I had breast-fed my babies, I was now nearly 52 and had not lost a limb or major organ in my mind! I did not want to be in hospital for more surgery and then have to worry about both sites healing properly and getting an infection. My husband fully supported my decision.

I can no longer wear my strappy dresses or low tops as I am concave in that area, so I wear round necked tops and have a falsie (that I can put in a bra/stick to my chest wall) to give me shape. Bras are difficult to find, but there are more important things to worry about!

Lisa's Story – Single Mastectomy with No Reconstruction

On 10th May 2017, I had a cyst diagnosed in my breast, and when a year later, in July 2018, I found another lump. I thought it was the same cyst that was now infected – so did my GP and Consultant. Unfortunately, it wasn't, and I was diagnosed with Triple Negative breast cancer, which presented as pain and a rapidly growing lump. Interestingly, after surgery, I was told that my tumour was sitting directly above the cyst - so in the same place. It would have been easy to assume it was just the cyst, so it's a good lesson in making sure to check things even if you think you know what's going on.

I was due to start a new job (I'm a nurse) and I had to speak to my employers and explain that I was having tests etc. They were fantastic, and even when I was diagnosed with cancer, they told me that wouldn't affect my employment with them.

Once treatment was underway, I had 6 cycles of chemotherapy (3 x FEC and 3 x T). On FEC, the tumour went from 52mm down to 3mm but then up to 22mm on Docetaxel. So, the Docetaxel was stopped, and it was decided to move to surgery. I had cancer in 2 nodes, but they responded to chemotherapy which was really good. It was also decided that after surgery and when I had healed, I would have more chemotherapy, Carboplatin, and then radiotherapy.

I had a radical mastectomy where they removed the pectoral muscles, the skin, breast tissue and lymph nodes. When I woke up from the surgery, I wasn't offered the chance to look at my scar, but I'm nosey, so within 10 minutes of being back in my room, I looked at my scar, and it was nice and neat. I was discharged the next day with a drain in place.

Unfortunately, after five days, the drain blocked, and fluid started leaking from where it was inserted, so I went to a clinic where they removed it. I then developed a seroma, and it grew so big I could hear it sloshing like a hot water bottle as I moved. From there, I had to have the area drained manually (with a needle that drew the fluid off) on quite a few occasions. It just wasn't healing, and two weeks later, the fluid broke through the wound and started leaking. I was given antibiotics to stop an infection, but as I'm a nurse, I knew something wasn't quite right, and so I kept going back to ask for it to be seen. Luckily during one of these visits, the surgeon came into the room to get something and saw my wound. He said it needed urgent attention because there was by now some necrotic tissue.

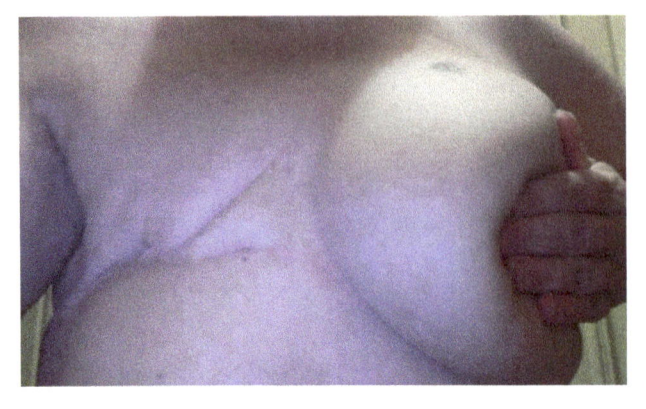

I saw the tissue viability team who treated the area, but it took over 14 weeks of visits every day to the clinic and daily dressing changes until it started to dry up and heal. During those 14 weeks, it was a long ordeal, and it often felt like we were going two steps forward and one step back.

My once neat scar now isn't as aesthetically pleasing, but I'm happy to live with it and don't want further surgery. I don't wear a bra or prosthetic and am a size FF on one side and flat on the other, but I wear whatever clothes I want, and I'm happy with how I am. I've also had a tattoo which is my jokey version of reconstruction, so I now have my "boobee" back.

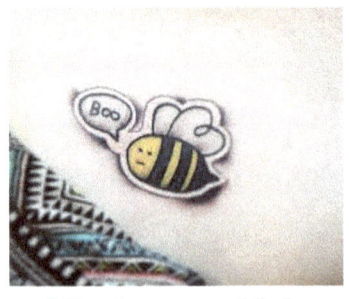

Jo's Story – Single Mastectomy with No Reconstruction

I was diagnosed on 7th December 2018 with a 20mm TNBC breast cancer in my right breast. The cancer was grade 2. Originally, I was told that I would have a lumpectomy, but after an MRI scan, a 7.4cm area of field change was found, so it was decided that I needed a mastectomy with a sentinel node biopsy. Fortunately, the sentinel node biopsy was clear.

I had surgery prior to chemotherapy, and I was told this meant that I would have to wait until after I had recovered from chemotherapy before reconstruction could be considered. I wasn't given the option of the immediate reconstruction as it was more important to my consultant that I could quickly recover from my surgery to start chemotherapy.

I did ask prior to surgery if I could have both removed, but again, my consultant said that he wanted to focus on removing cancer, which I thought was a good idea.

I had my surgery at the end of January 2019, and it went well. I was out the following day and, after a couple of weeks, was recovered. In March, I started my chemotherapy. Four rounds of EC and then twelve weeks of Paclitaxel and Carboplatin. I finally completed all active treatment in September 2019.

A few months after, I asked if I could go ahead with a second mastectomy, and I was offered information about reconstruction. I have always known I didn't want reconstruction, as to me, the surgery sounded horrible, and I didn't see the point. I hate being a uni-boober, though and kept asking for a second mastectomy for symmetry. After a few false starts and over a year after my active treatment was completed, I finally got put on the surgeon's list for this in February 2021. However, I think I am in for a long wait, as it has already been another year on, and I have heard nothing.

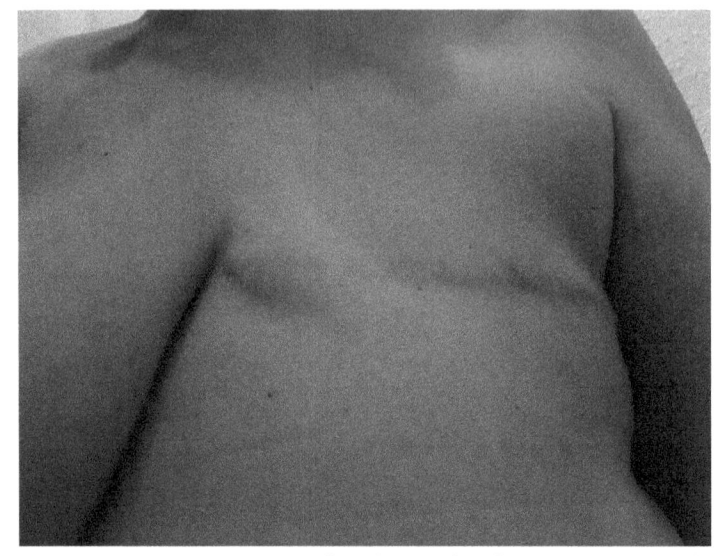

Reconstruction is completely right for some people, but for me, I would prefer to go flat. I can still wear my false boobs if I want a bit of shape, but it seems much more comfortable and appealing to me not to have to worry about bras all the time!

CHAPTER 18

RADIOTHERAPY

Of all the cancer treatments, radiotherapy is probably the easiest, but the side effects can be tough because your body has already gone through chemotherapy and surgery, and now you're going to have Star Wars of the chest. It all sounds very daunting, but let's look at the process you'll probably go through.

The first stage of radiotherapy is a planning appointment. This can take anything from 30 minutes to 2 hours. During this appointment, you will have a scan, (different departments use different scans), but it's normally a CT scan with, or without, contrast (a dye that's injected into your arm). The reason for this is that the radiotherapy team need to make sure they have the exact location of your tumour, tumour site, chest wall and/or nodes that need to be zapped!

To ensure they can line you up to the exact position for the radiotherapy beams, you will have between 1 and 5 tiny black pinpoint tattoos put on your breast. The tattoo placement is critical because it means each appointment will be faster as the tattoo marks are used to direct the radiotherapy beams to the exact place the treatment is needed, so there's no need for lengthy appointments each visit.

Depending on your diagnosis, you will either have radiotherapy to just your tumour area or your tumour and node area (if the nodes had cancer in them), and in the case of some ladies where perhaps they've had a mastectomy, the whole breast may be treated with or without the chest wall etc.

For some ladies, especially if they have larger breasts, or are finding it difficult to stay still, a cast may be made of the chest area, which will then be placed across the breast area at each appointment.

By now, in your breast cancer timeframe, you're probably used to having your breasts out for consultants, nurses etc., and I'm afraid it will be the same with radiotherapy. Just bear in mind that this is their everyday job, and nothing they see will shock them. The embarrassment is probably more for you than them, but the team will understand this and are normally incredibly kind and make you feel comfortable.

You will most probably have to have either one or both arms above your head, and this can be difficult if you're still stiff from surgery. It's imperative that you do the exercises your breast care team gave you after surgery to help regain flexibiity. The more you do this (once healed, of course), the less likely you are to have trouble with the radiotherapy.

If you are having treatment to your left breast, the other thing you may be asked to do is to hold your breath for up to 20 seconds (usually shorter, but if you plan for 20 seconds, you'll have it covered). What this does is move your heart away from the area that's having radiotherapy. Whether you're asked to do this, or not, depends on the type of equipment being used and also the specific location of your tumour. So you can prepared (just in case), it's a really good idea to practice holding your breath in the run-up to your treatment. If you have a cold or cough or anything to do with your breathing, this can be problematic, so please make sure you talk to your team so they can plan accordingly.

Radiotherapy appointments are typically Monday to Friday with the weekends off, and you'll either have an intense dose regime of 5 days (which is becoming more popular now), or you may have daily appointments spanning a 3 or 5-week timeframe (again, every day Monday to Friday). Your hospital will advise how long your course will be.

During treatment, you lie on your back and once in place, the team will leave the room to take several measurements using X-rays and other equipment to ensure you're in the right place. At all points, they can hear you talk, so although you're in the room on your own, if you need to talk to them, you can. They do ask that you remain very still, though.

Once the machine starts, you will hear whirring and beeping, but nothing touches you. Apart from the sounds, you won't be aware that anything is happening. At certain points, your team may speak to you to give instructions over an intercom (such as when to hold your breath and then breathe normally again).

Although you will have a dose of radiation, you won't be radioactive, so there's no need to take any extra precautions.

Side Effects

Changes to Skin Appearance

Radiotherapy works in a way that the beam hits the spot that's being targeted, but because it doesn't hit a solid structure, it will hit the spot and then travel past it. Normally this will be limited by the dose you're given, but if your tumour is towards the back of your breast, you may find that you have a sore patch on your back towards the end of treatment. This can look a bit like sunburn.

During treatment, if your skin changes in colour or texture, please speak to your team. They will often ask you to make sure you moisturise the area really well before, during, and after treatment. Radiotherapy can cause the skin to tighten, redden and become very sore, so it's important to take good care of that area. Not everybody reacts in this way, and some may just feel only minor discomfort, but others may need a bit more care. Your radiotherapy team can advise on the best creams to use (so please make sure you ask at your planning appointment). They may even give you cream. A pad soaked in the cream can also give relief if you have just a small area that you want to treat.

Other creams that people have used are Double Base Gel and Aloe Vera. Combining the two and putting some in the fridge (definitely not freezer) and using it when it's a bit cold can help with the heat but please be careful with this. You don't want the cream to be so cold that it causes your skin to burn. Skin redness usually settles within 2-4 weeks of treatment ending, but if it's ongoing, you must see your team.

Towards the end of treatment, skin can also break down – this can happen where you have a scar or if your tumour is closer to the skin. You must tell your team because they will be able to give you specific dressings to put on top.

If you can, allow your skin to breathe – it may be worth not wearing clothes on your top half when you're at home. I appreciate this may not be possible, but if you can, it will help. Just don't open the door to the postman!

Tiredness and Weakness

This side effect is often a shock and not expected. It can creep up on you the longer the treatments go on. Unfortunately, tiredness can continue for weeks after treatment has finished. Rest when you need to, but studies have shown gentle exercise during and after treatment may help combat tiredness, but I appreciate you may just feel like you want to curl up on the sofa with a good book! Do what feels right for you.

Swelling of the Breast

Radiotherapy can interfere with the breast's natural drainage via the lymphatic system, and if you've already had a seroma or issues after surgery, you may be prone to this. It happens infrequently, but if it does happen, it can be very uncomfortable. It normally resolves a few weeks after treatment has stopped, but if it doesn't, then you may be referred to the lymphoedema clinic and possibly have some specialist massages to encourage the area to drain.

Loss of Hair to Armpit

Your armpit hair may not have returned after chemotherapy, but if it has, it may fall out again. I suspect that for many ladies, this would be a welcome side effect! It will grow back in most cases, though.

Restricted Movements to Arm and Shoulder

This is fairly common and can get worse with the longer treatments to go on. This is a direct result of the changes that your skin is undergoing, and it's not just the tumour and nodes blasted with radiotherapy. Your muscles are also in the same area. Your team may suggest some physiotherapy to help give you better movement. Please ask and don't suffer in silence if this is happening to you.

Long Term Side Effects and Complications

Unfortunately, as with lots of cancer treatments, there can be long term side effects. The most common is a change in the shape and texture of the breast. It's very common for a radiated breast to appear smaller than your other breast, and this can be a gradual change and can continue for a number of years.

There are also other complications that can occur, but they're very rare such as heart or bone issues and breathing problems. I need to stress that these are rare, but they do happen. If you don't feel well, please see your team so they can assess if radiotherapy has caused an issue or whether it could be unrelated.

If you have had a mastectomy and reconstruction with implants and then had radiotherapy, there is a chance that the radiotherapy has (or will) damage the implants. This is unfortunately very common, and it's why having implants and radiotherapy are not recommended. There are ways to avoid this happening, and if you want implants, please speak to your surgeon to see what can be done.

Because changes to your skin and breast area can continue for a few years after radiotherapy, it's advised to keep moisturising as much as possible and for as long as possible.

For most ladies, radiotherapy will pass easily with only minimal discomfort. Many choose to work through this part of the treatment and, apart from feeling tired, find it very doable. If you've chosen to work through treatment but find tiredness is becoming a problem, please take some time off if possible. Don't forget your body needs its energy to heal.

CHAPTER 19

HAIR

All about Hair

Some ladies don't mind losing their hair and feel it's liberating. I wasn't one of them, and losing my hair made me feel very self-conscious, old, and generally miserable. It seems so unfair that you're diagnosed with cancer, and then the treatment makes you look different, but that's the reality. Some ladies want to hide their diagnosis, telling people only when they want to, or they have younger children and want to remain looking "the same". There's no right or wrong way to how you feel about losing your hair, but if hair loss is something you are worried about, there are things that you can do to make yourself feel better and even try to keep your hair, and I'll address these later in this chapter.

When Will I Lose My Hair?

A typical timescale for when hair starts to shed is around the beginning of your second cycle of chemotherapy (if you're on a three-week regime). So, it may start anywhere between days 17 to 23. An indicator that it's starting is a very strange feeling of ants crawling over your scalp in hobnail boots! I really don't have a better descriptor than that, but it can be really sore. What you're actually feeling are the hair follicles dying off and struggling with the weight of your hair, but for some reason, your team may not prepare you for this.

If you've chosen to shave your hair off, this is the perfect time to do it because you will get almost immediate relief. Please be careful because you don't want to cut your head as this can then cause infections. If you have access to some clippers, you may want to use those. In my experience, hairdressers will usually do this for you for free. There's no need to go totally bald at this stage, so you can just take it to around a few millimetres which will still give you coverage if you'd prefer.

Hair on your head is normally the first to go, followed by body hair and then lastly, your eyebrows and eyelashes. Some ladies are really lucky and don't lose their eyebrows or eyelashes. My brows and lashes hung on for about 10 weeks before they finally gave up and made a swift exit! A strange thing that may happen is you'll also lose nasal hair – it wasn't something I had even considered when I thought of body hair.

Cold Capping

A company called Paxman have developed a system that, in some cases, may help you to keep all, or some, of your hair during chemotherapy. This is called "cold capping" and involves wearing a multi-layered helmet on your head that is temperature controlled to between -15 to -40F. How this works is that the cold repels the chemotherapy and protects the hair follicles from being attacked (that's a very basic explanation, but I hope it gives you an idea). A concern for some ladies is that it may stop the chemotherapy from getting everywhere, and in tests carried out by Paxman, they state the risk is very small. If you're worried, please speak with your oncologist to get his or her opinion.

On a practical basis, Paxman says that you will lose some hair and for cold capping to be considered a success, you won't have to wear a wig, scarf, hat, or any other hair cover.

Since 2016 when I used the cold cap, Paxman has updated their website, and they have published the following results as an indication of what may be possible. However, they point out that these are examples, and no two people are the same. For some, cold capping works amazingly well. For others, they lose a good amount of hair but can still disguise it and not wear a wig and then for others, they lose more hair, and it's problematic to hide:

Taxanes
We see great success with taxanes, around 70-80% chance of keeping 50% of your hair.

70 to
80%

Anthracyclines
We see success with anthracyclines, around a 35-40% chance of keeping 50% of your hair.

35 to
40%

Docetaxel
We see a 75% chance of keeping 50% of your hair with docetaxel, but scalp cooling also mitigates the risk of persistent alopecia

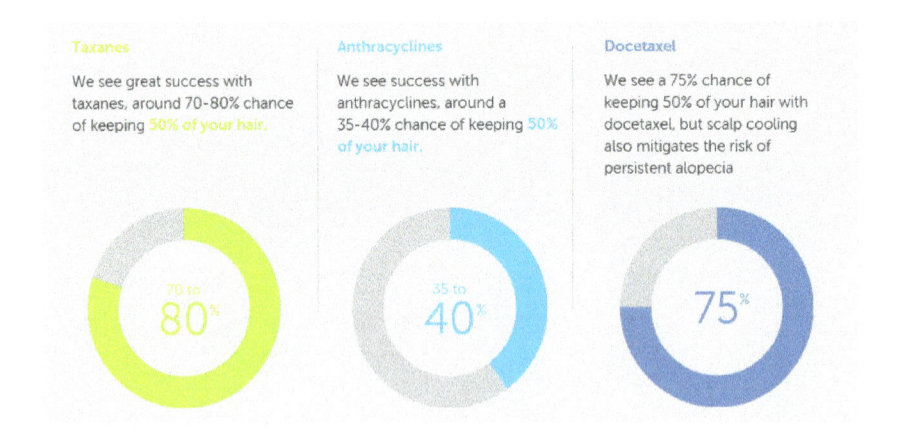

75%

Image replicated with the kind permission of Paxman Scalp Cooling
www.coldcap.com.

As a reminder, Taxanes include Paclitaxel, but as you can see, there's a separate box above for Docetaxel, and this is because it's known to be more aggressive on hair during treatment. Anthracyclines include FEC, EC and AC. Although the above doesn't have Carboplatin listed, there is a decision-making tool on their website, and you can find out more there. Also missing from the list is Capecitabine which you may remember from earlier chapters as the drug in tablet form given after radiotherapy to some but not all. You don't often lose your hair with this chemotherapy, so cold capping wouldn't be advised with this drug, and as you take it at home, it would be impossible to administer the cold cap.

Depending on the type of chemotherapy drug you're having, you have to wear the cold cap for around 30 minutes before treatment, during treatment and then for about an hour after. For me, the cold cap had to stay on for at least 3-3.5 hours with EC, and it's important that in order for it to work, it must stay on for the recommended length of time for the specific chemotherapy you're having. Your nurses will know what's right, and certainly, on the Paxman machine, there's normally a leaflet attached giving all the timings.

When you first decide to use a cold cap, your breast care nurse will fit you for an inner cap (it's rubber, and it's the bit that generates the cold next to your scalp). There are several sizes, and it's imperative to get a very tight fit all over the cap. The most common area that's difficult to fit is the very top/crown of the cap.

Over the top of the inner cap, you have what looks like a soft cycling helmet to hold everything in place - and this has a chin strap that ensures good contact with the scalp. During cold capping, I looked like Tutankhamun because I found a soft piece of fabric that I hooked under the chin strap so I could pull it down to stop some of the choking feelings that the tightness of the chin strap can cause. It looked like a very fetching Egyptian beard! Because it can be challenging to get a good fit, I've noticed that it's becoming common for ladies to purchase exercise bands to pull the top of the cap down during treatment to ensure it meets the crown.

Once the outer helmet is put on, the whole unit is hooked up to the Paxman machine that maintains temperature throughout the treatment. The first 15 minutes of wearing the cap really are the worse, and for some, it does become unbearable. For others, after the initial feeling of wanting to rip it off, it becomes much easier (and I even managed to fall asleep with it on)! You will probably be advised to take a painkiller 30 minutes before you put the cap on, but please check with your nurse, who can advise what to take and when.

Because you're being turned into a human icicle, you may want to wear lots of warm clothing and have a blanket over you. I had on 5 layers and those included cold-weather underwear suitable for skiing. I never felt cold (apart from my head), but it's advisable to wrap up in as many layers as you can.

For me, cold capping didn't really work, unfortunately. I started to lose my hair around day 18 after my first cycle of EC. My scalp started to fizz and become painful, but this can happen with ladies who have success, so I ploughed on. I did everything I was supposed to do - I only washed my hair once a week in tepid water, I didn't brush it with a normal hairbrush, only a tangle teezer, I didn't dry it with a hairdryer, straighten, or apply any products. I religiously stuck to the Paxman rules, but unfortunately, it didn't work.

Normal hair loss (without chemotherapy is around 100 hairs per day), so you will always see some hair loss, and with cold capping, you not only lose the 100 hairs but then hair loss over and above that. The hair doesn't come out in huge chunks, but if you run your hands through your hair, you'll find hair each time you do it. Some days the loss is better than others, but the amount you lose is totally individual.

For me, by the end of my 4th cycle of EC, the hair on my crown was the thinnest area, although overall, it was thin, limp and a bit stringy looking. It's difficult to estimate, but I think I probably lost at least 50% of my hair and was so self-conscious that at this point, I was wearing a wig over the hair I had left. On average, every day, I was losing hair that could be bundled up and filled my palm – about the size of a tennis ball. It was alarming how much there was on a daily basis, and it's surprising how much we can lose but still have a lot of hair on our heads! A nasty side effect is that hair was everywhere – every room in the house, over my clothes, bedclothes and you couldn't escape hair so be warned you'll be hoovering more than normal!

I think the reason my crown thinned so much was that my first cold cap was fitted by a junior nurse with little training, and, in hindsight, the fit wasn't great, and because the crown was not in direct contact with the cold cap, I lost most of the hair there. Another area that thinned was around my face and ears, and this is quite common as the cap doesn't always fit exactly.

Whilst the cold cap only partly worked for me, I have seen some ladies who have had remarkable results. There doesn't seem to be a way to guarantee to limit the hair loss, but the things the ladies have done in common have been to not just dampen the hair before putting on the cap but to totally saturate it (which makes sense as there's more to freeze) and the cap has been a really good fit. Other than that, I think it's just down to luck.

Don't forget the downside is that each chemotherapy session will be considerably longer than if you don't want to cold cap (up to 2 hours longer or more), so you may want to consider this. If you have weekly chemotherapy, this can also be a bit daunting, but I'm afraid there's no other solution.

It's definitely worth trying, and you can stop at any time if it's not working, or you really can't bear it. Of course, if you stop, your hair will be lost as if you're not cold capped.

Would I cold cap again? Yes, I would. I gave up after my 4th EC because my hair looked so terrible, and I was wearing a wig in any case that it seemed silly putting myself through any more sessions. Also, I was due to have 12 weekly Paclitaxel sessions, and I just couldn't see how my hair was going to look any better. With Paclitaxel, it is less aggressive on your hair, so the chances are, I wouldn't have lost as much, but I just didn't want to go through that.

A very weird side effect for me was that I couldn't bear the smell of the freezer sections in supermarkets. I have no idea why because the cold cap doesn't smell at all, but I couldn't go anywhere near the freezers!

A huge benefit for me with cold capping is that I think it did give me some protection because when chemotherapy finally ended, my hair grew back SO quickly! My hairdresser was really surprised at how fast it came back. By 8 weeks, I had between 3-and 5cm of growth! Of course, it may have grown back at that speed anyway, but I do think cold capping helped.

Nasal Hair!

Nasal hair – who knew this even had a purpose! Well, it's there for a reason, and when it's gone, you may find that your nose drips without you being aware of it! It's such a strange sensation but don't be alarmed. You're not leaking – this is normal! Once the hair leaves, there's nothing to tell you that your nose is dripping because you lose the sensation! There's no cure (other than having a tissue on hand), but as soon as the hair grows back, this will resolve.

Eyelashes

When your eyelashes depart, you may find that your eyes are really sore and stream uncontrollably. Strangely this is called dry eye syndrome! Your GP or pharmacist can suggest lubricating eye drops that will help. On occasion, the drops won't work, but there are lots of brands to try, so if one doesn't stop your symptoms, try another.

One other thing that caught me by surprise was when my eyelashes came back. About a month afterwards, they all fell out again at the same time. I was so worried they weren't going to come back, but they did. This happened to me three times. What causes this is when hair grows, it grows in cycles, and normally each hair has its own cycle, so as one eyelash is growing, another is dying off and falling out. However, when you lose all your eyelashes from chemotherapy, you lose them all at the same time, and the growth cycle stops. When they start growing again, they all start growing around the same time, so it follows that they will also fall out at the same time. For some people (like me), this was very noticeable, but for others, less so. It will stabilise as the growth cycles establish and change, and you'll suddenly notice that you have all your eyelashes back and they haven't disappeared for a while.

False Eyelashes

When you lose your eyelashes, especially if you've worn makeup for most of your adult life, you may feel you look different. Unfortunately, there's no magic answer to this other than to use false eyelashes. There are so many brands, and it can be daunting if you've not worn them before. I bought about 30 pairs (a very expensive business) before I found a brand that not only looked natural but felt comfortable. I found Eylure to be the best brand for me, but I did try ones specifically for chemotherapy (they felt heavy and looked odd, which was a shame) and magnetic ones that attach to an eyeliner – that was a disaster, and I looked like a witch!

You do need to experiment, but the one thing I found that made this easier (and if I wear falsies, I use this still) is an eyelash applicator. It looks a bit like an eyelash curler, and you can pick them up for under £10. They hold the eyelash so you can concentrate on getting the lash in the right place. What works for you won't work for the next person, so this is one area that you will have to experiment with if you want to wear eyelashes,

I'm allergic to most types of glue (although, in fairness, I didn't try the Eylure glue), but I found an American company called Thrive Cosmetics which has a range of makeup for patients undergoing chemotherapy that takes out most of the nasties in normal cosmetics. I bought their glue which was amazing, but it took ages to arrive in the post and was hideously expensive. Unfortunately, at the current time, they are not shipping to the UK, but I'm sure those restrictions will be lifted soon, and it may be worth looking at their website.

A good, long-lasting eyeliner can also give your eyes a wider look if you normally wear makeup. I preferred the waterproof, long-lasting variety because my eyes used to stream as mentioned above and my favourite product is called Eye of Horus and can be found if you search the internet. At the time of writing, it's around £20, so a bit pricey, but it lasted me for at least 6 months, wearing it every day, and once it's on, it doesn't budge – great if you have watery eyes!

Eyebrows

I've already mentioned in the chapter of things to do before treatment starts that having your brows microbladed is a really good idea. However, there are alternatives.

Even though I had my brows microbladed because I couldn't have the top up before treatment started, I used Wunderbrow to just give a bit more colour. Wunderbrow (and I'm sure there are other similar products) is waterproof and smudge-proof, so if you go into the rain, your brows won't slide down your face! This product is a liquid with a brush, and so long as you keep the cap on at all times, it can be used for months. I found that to use it so it looked natural, I would wipe the brush against the rim of the tube to remove most of the liquid and then I would use the end of the brush to stipple onto my brows (rather than use it in a sweeping motion). The stippling gave a more natural look. However, if you need a fuller look, you will need to use a swiping motion.

There are also stick-on brows and also stencils that you can use to give the illusion of brows and give you a natural shape. These will need some practice to make sure you get them in the right place and are not too heavy-handed, but this may be a solution if you want to try everything.

Alternative Head Wear

Even if you decide to rock the no-hair look, you may need to invest in some headwear because in the winter, your head may get horribly cold, and the feel of rain on your head is very strange indeed – none of that will be new to bald men, but I was surprised at how cold my head did get. In bed at night, your head may also get chilly, so a soft beanie can be a good idea. In the summer, you will need to protect your scalp from the sun, so something light but giving coverage is recommended.

If you're looking at different types of headwear, there are quite a few options:

- Scarves – you can learn to use normal scarves, and if you look on YouTube, there are lots of ideas on how to tie them. I've got to say that I tried this, but rather than looking like a glamorous 50s housewife, I looked like an Egyptian mummy that had been tied up by a trainee! Some scarves, specifically for chemotherapy patients, are more shaped and can be less challenging, so when tied correctly, they can really look good and can be combined with hairpieces.

- Hairpieces that look like fringes or ponytails can be attached to scarves and hats, and just having a bit of hair on the show can give the illusion of a full head of hair.

- Turbans – you can tie material yourself (again, have a look on YouTube for how to do this), or you can buy ready-made turbans that have an adjustable band inside to keep things secure.

- Hats and Beanies – There are so many different styles available but wearing a beanie may keep you cosy. If you buy one specifically made for chemotherapy/hair loss patients, you'll find that it doesn't have any labels or seams to irritate. If you buy a normal beanie, be aware of this and check for comfort before buying.

- Wigs – I'm going to write more about wigs in the next section.

- There are quite a few websites for headwear specifically made for chemotherapy patients, and you'll find links in chapter 30.

Wigs

Years ago, wearing wigs was something only older men and women might have, and they were sometimes very obvious. Thankfully, wearing wigs has become much more acceptable, and lots of young people use them as fashion statements!

Never in a million years did I think I would get used to wearing a wig! It's funny how things change!

If you have breast cancer, you either qualify for a discount voucher (some hospitals give them to you - others don't) of around £100 and/or you might be eligible to have the VAT removed when you buy from a shop. I've never been given a voucher, but I filled in a form at my local wig shop (I didn't even know there was such a thing beforehand!) and that entitled me to buy at a pre-VAT price.

Some hospitals have links to shops that supply wigs or even have a salon within the hospital, but your breast care nurse will be able to tell you what's available. I actually found a wig shop near to me that was fantastic, so I was able to go and try them on, but I also found some really cheap wigs on Amazon that were surprisingly "un-wig" like and were really good buy (under £30!).

How to Buy a Wig:

Before starting treatment, I went to the wig shop and tried on several wigs, but my heart wasn't really in it. I bought a blonde, long bob - similar to how I'd just had my hair cut - but I didn't really concentrate on how it was made or how it would actually feel when worn all day. Also, as I still had hair, the wig didn't sit flat on my scalp, so I couldn't see what the real effect would be. Consequently, it stayed in the box and only made an appearance when I realised looking like Albert Einstein wasn't really acceptable in public! When I put it on, I realised my mistake. It was ok, but it was at the cheaper end of the market, and the parting really did look "wiggy".

As my hair was looking awful during cold capping, and with the encouragement of a friend, I went back to the shop to give wigs another chance. By the way, ALWAYS take a friend with you if you can. It's difficult to be objective and know what looks good if you're on your own although the staff are incredibly kind and very knowledgeable, a second and third opinion is always good.

Before I went, I looked online at the various different styles but decided that I wanted to look almost like I did pre-chemotherapy as I wanted to look as much like me as possible. I tried on tons of wigs! You'll probably be surprised at what you end up buying! Although I've had long hair all my life, it never occurred to me to buy one with long hair! I have no idea why! Anyway, I tried on a long one just out of interest and was so pleased I did.

Some people want to have a completely different style, length or colour and are quite happy to have a few different ones (purple for Monday, blue for Tuesday, ginger for Wednesday etc.), but for me, I wanted something that looked fairly natural.

The construction of a wig varies quite considerably. They can be heavy, lightweight, have a breathable interior, have a realistic parting, hair darker at the roots and with different subtle colours to give a realistic look. They can be made of human hair or be synthetic. Some can be styled with gentle heat, and others can't, but they each have different tightening mechanisms on the inside to adjust the fit. There's so much to learn!

Human hair wigs are more expensive than synthetic ones, and they have to be looked after slightly differently, but synthetic wigs have come a long way in terms of construction, so they are far less likely to have the shiny hair look that you may remember if you've had a Sindy or Barbie doll.

Wig Caps

To wear a wig successfully and to stop it from slipping, you will need a wig cap. These can be bought online and are normally around £1-2 each, sometimes less. They look a bit like a pair of tights (obviously without the legs!) with a wide rim that goes around the edge of your head and face. The purpose of a wig cap is to keep any hair you have, flattened to your head, so the wig fits properly, but without hair, it also stops the wig from moving around. There are various types of wig caps, so experiment to see which one suits you best. One thing to mention is that you may want to buy quite a few of these because they will need washing every day (or at least every other day) as they do absorb oils from your head.

Interestingly, when you first put on a wig (especially if you haven't got any hair, it's very easy to pull it too far forward on your forehead. Too far forward can look very strange. A tip I saw on YouTube was to put your wig on and then ease it back a bit. Stand in front of a mirror and do this. If you have a mobile phone, take some photos, and look at them objectively – does the wig look in the right place? The other thing you can do (but this requires preparation and needs to be done before you lose your hair, is to get a ruler and measure from the centre of your eye upwards to wear your natural hairline is. Don't use your eyebrows because don't forget; they will go too. You'll soon find that wearing a wig is easy and second nature, but in the first few weeks, you'll be fiddling around to get it right.

What to Look For in a Wig

The first one I bought had quite a heavy interior, and it wasn't as comfortable as subsequent ones I bought, and I quickly learnt that I wanted a more natural look and fit.

The best wig I bought had a lace front with a lightweight and breathable monofilament top. When you look at a wig, the front that frames the face and the partings can be giveaways that it's not your natural hair. The lace front gives a really natural look to the front of the wig (see photo). You'll see that it's very hard to see it's a wig – but it is! I also had a fringe cut into my wig because (a) I normally have a fringe and (b) IF the wig doesn't have a lace front, a good way of disguising the front area is to hide it behind a fringe. Please don't attempt to cut the wig yourself. In order to look natural, they need to be cut by a hairdresser or the wig shop staff who are trained to do this.

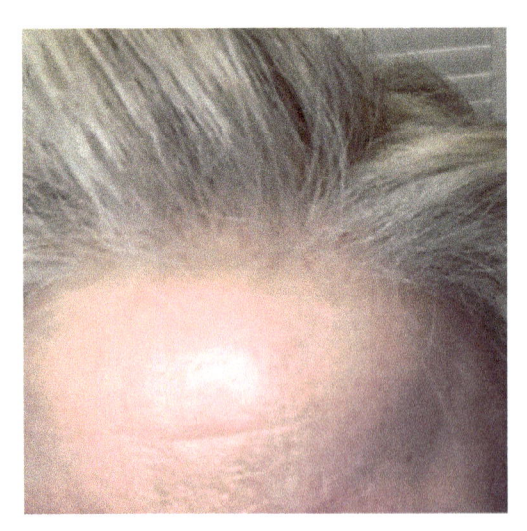

In the next photo, you'll see the interior of the wig. The lace front is at the top of the photo, and you can see that there's only a thin piece of fabric under the hair – this is what gives it a natural look because your scalp shows through the material.

Halfway up the photo, on either side, you'll see slightly wider edge pieces. These are the bits that go around your ears, and they act as a really good guide, so you know that it's in place.

The monofilament crown, in this photo, looks bulky but isn't. It's soft and very pliable. Again, you can see your scalp through it, although not to the extent of the lace front.

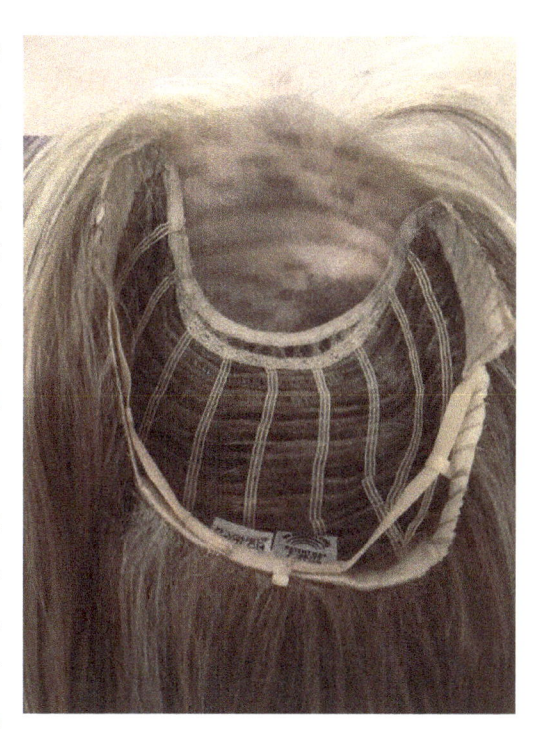

At the bottom of the photo, there are two small straps on the inside rim. The strap on the right-hand side is perhaps easier to see. At the end of each strap, there's a piece of Velcro used to tighten the wig when it's in place. Wigs have different ways to tighten them, so have a good look at the inside to see how to fasten yours. You may need to experiment to get the best fit for you.

Some wigs can be styled with straighteners on a low setting, but please check because not all can. Also, my wig could be parted on either side or in the middle, and some wigs can, others can't.

Wearing a wig gave me so much confidence and made me feel "normal". Unless I told people I was going through cancer treatment, I could hide it fairly well, and that was important to me. This is a personal choice, and I love seeing ladies who have the confidence to go bald one of my friends used to wear a different colour wig each week, and I loved that too! Whatever you choose to do, it'll be right for you.

Taking Care of Your Wig:

For prolonging the life of your wig, it's important to follow the instructions that come with it. For example, you should never brush it with a normal brush. Either use one specially made for wigs or a Tangle Teezer.

Especially with longer wigs, with constant wear, the ends can start to feel a bit woolly and may fan out, looking a bit like candy floss. There's no way to avoid this, and if all else fails, it's a good idea to have the ends nibbled off by a hairdresser to keep it looking good. Obviously, it won't grow back, so go easy on this! However, I did learn a neat trick, and you may want to read the next few paragraphs before running for the scissors.

Even if you wash the wig (and you should wash it at least once every two weeks in specialist wig shampoo and leave-in conditioner), it won't get rid of the frizz/clumpiness. I watched tons of online videos about wig care, and most of them said to steam the wig, so I bought a little hand steamer, and yes, it worked, but not 100%.

I then found the most fantastic video on YouTube where a hairdresser literally poured boiling hot water through the wig (clearly not when wearing it but over the sink, being careful not to scold), and I'm not sure why it works, but it does! I boiled a full kettle, held my wig over the sink and poured the hot water over the hair, concentrating on the clumpy bits and then smoothed in a small amount of leave-in wig conditioner and rinsed it very lightly, again in the boiling hot water. I brushed it with a Tangle Teezer and then laid it on a towel to dry and couldn't believe my eyes! It actually looked better than when I bought it! If you start to see the frizziness on the ends, it's worth trying this trick to see if it helps.

Drying your wig should be done lying flat. Don't be tempted to dry on a mannequin head or wig stand because this can pull the wig out of shape, and also, if it's a polystyrene head, it can also take much longer to dry. Gently place the wig on a towel, and with another towel, dab off as much excess water as you can and then leave to air-dry. If you use a hairdryer, you will shorten the life of the wig, so leave it to air-dry whenever possible. It may be that you want to buy two wigs so you can still have one to wear when the other is being washed.

Wig Stands

I found a wig stand really useful. You can buy different types, but you really only need a plastic one that folds away. These are inexpensive and are shaped like a head. It's a good idea, when not wearing the wig, to allow it to breathe and hold its shape, and that's where the wig stand comes in.

What About After Treatment Ends?

Hair Extensions / Systems

If you've always had long hair, you may be impatient for your hair to grow and for you to have lovely long hair again. When your hair gets to about 5-6cm long, you might be able to have extensions. There is a company called Racoon Hair in Recovery that specialises in extensions for clients who lose their hair because of treatments or alopecia. The difference with their extensions is the way they attach the extension to the hair, which uses a kinder method and glue. Your hair does have to be a certain length before this is possible because the extensions need to hold on to something. Also, don't forget that your hair may be weak when it first starts to come through, so it's best to wait until you have the right length. Extensions are an expensive business, but they can give you so much confidence that you may be prepared to spend the money. I had extensions put in, and for the first few months, my short hair would stick out a bit and be obvious to me (but probably not to anybody else). As my hair grew longer, it merged with the extensions, and you really couldn't tell I had them in.

There are alternative systems to extensions, ones that use hairpieces that are semi-permanent. They are fitted with glue that attaches around the edges of your hairline but still allows your natural hair to grow back underneath. You can even go swimming in them (although I'm not sure I would be brave enough to do that)!

It's definitely worth investigating the alternatives but make sure that they're safe – perhaps do some research and get in touch with other cancer patients who may have tried the system you're looking at.

Colouring Your Hair

If you ask an oncologist, "When can I dye my hair" they will tell you 6 months from your last chemotherapy. That's a very long time to wait if your hair has come back grey and you hate it, or it's come back another colour (which can also happen)! The reason for the wait is that your hair will still be weak from the chemotherapy and all hair dyes have "nasties" in them. Some are worse than others. Typically, the darker they are, the more prone they are to cause reactions.

There are a number of hair dye brands that have removed "most" of the nasties. It's impossible to take them all out because they simply wouldn't work. In my experience, if you want to dye your hair a darker colour, brown, black, or even a dark red, it's possible to get some very nice dyes from a natural range. However, if you want to go blonde, it's much more challenging. I'm not sure why but it could be because they're less pigmented. Most "natural" dyes are semi-permanent, so they will wash out after a few washes. If you want to try one, please look on the internet for suggestions or ask in any groups you may belong to. Products are being launched all the time but make sure you look at the ingredients to check they really are free from nasties!

CHAPTER 20

BISPHOSPHONATES

As we've already explored, unlike hormonal breast cancer, there are limited options that can help prevent a Triple Negative breast cancer from returning. However, for naturally post-menopausal ladies (and I emphasise the word "natural" rather than chemotherapy-induced menopause), there is one option. This is called bisphosphonate therapy.

The use of Bisphosphonates in a breast cancer setting was the subject of a 5-year study in Japan, where they discovered that giving bisphosphonates to naturally post-menopausal women helped to strengthen bones, reduced bone breakdown and potentially created a barrier against secondary bone cancer. The reason that this is very rarely given to pre-menopausal ladies (unless there's an underlying medical condition or other reason) is that pre-menopausal bones are normally strong enough, and it's the bone density that is lost as we age which leaves us potentially susceptible to a cancer attack.

So, whilst bisphosphonates don't work in the same way as treatment tablets for ladies with hormonal breast cancer, studies indicate that they do give some protection against secondary bone cancer. Interestingly, the "Predict" tool that oncologists use to predict life expectancy/prognosis for ladies with breast cancer shows that having bisphosphonates can increase your chances of survival by 2%. That doesn't sound a lot, but it's better than 0%, and every little bit helps!

Bisphosphonates have become more popular in the past 5 years, and the majority of post-menopausal women will be offered them. It does have to be taken as soon as treatment finishes/within 3 months, so if you haven't been offered it and you fit the criteria, speak to your oncologist. Because it's at the tail end of treatment and a bolt-on, it can be occasionally overlooked.

There are several different methods of giving bisphosphonates to patients, but the most common are:

- 6 monthly infusions. A clear liquid is administered via a regular cannula normally in the back of your hand. The infusion takes approximately 15 minutes, but there may be a further 15 minutes to have an infusion of saline before and after that acts as a "flush". Typically, you also have a blood test a few days before just to check your liver, kidney, and red blood cell levels.

Or

- A tablet is taken regularly (normally daily). Sometimes this tablet is given first, but if it can't be tolerated, you may be moved on to the infusions.

The most commonly used bisphosphonate drugs are:

- Alendronate (Binosto, Fosamax)
- Ibandronate (Boniva)

- Risedronate (Actonel, Atelvia)

- Zoledronic acid (Reclast, Zometa)

You can get side effects with bisphosphonates, and the most common is 'flu-like symptoms and tiredness, which are normally short-lived. Typically, side effects will be worse with the first infusion but lessen with each one after that. Like all other drugs, there is a long list of side effects, but generally, it is well tolerated. Some ladies find that the second infusion may give them side effects but as these only last a few days and are every 6 months (if having infusions), it is usually tolerated well. Tablets tend to have fewer side effects.

Ironically, bisphosphonates can lower calcium and vitamin D levels, so sometimes it's suggested you take daily supplements to replace any deficiency, but this must be discussed with your oncologist as vitamins and minerals can interfere with other drugs you may be taking.

The major risk of having bisphosphonate treatment is jawbone necrosis. The risk is very, very small, and it's usually where dental work is compromised before starting treatment and not rectified. So, prior to starting bisphosphonates, you MUST see your dentist and have any dental work required, such as extractions, fillings etc. Your oral health must be good. Otherwise, it will be a risk to commence bisphosphonate therapy. Some hospitals will now insist you see a dentist, and your oral health is signed off before they will even contemplate giving you this treatment. The one issue with this is that getting a dental appointment (if you're not already registered with a dentist) can be cost-prohibitive, but you may be referred to a dental hospital. Please see the chapter on teeth for more information.

CHAPTER 21

TEETH

You may wonder why there's a chapter dedicated to teeth in a book about breast cancer, and prior to my diagnosis, I would have said the same thing. Because teeth are looked after by Dentists rather than Doctors, they are often overlooked after a cancer diagnosis, but they are as important to your health as any other part of your body and in fact, with chemotherapy and radiotherapy, you need to be extra vigilant because complications can arise.

Hopefully, you will have been advised to visit your dentist prior to treatment start, and one of the reasons for this is that during chemotherapy, your dentist may be reluctant to do any work required because of the risk of infection. During chemotherapy and radiotherapy, you are immunosuppressed, i.e., your immune system is less able to fight off infection. Also, if you need an extraction, for example, healing can take much longer.

That's not the only reason, though. Your mouth is the gateway to your body, so during treatment, you want to minimise any type of infection. You may think there's not too much of an issue if your mouth isn't in tip-top condition, but it is. You could lose your teeth, and I don't say that lightly.

Why Can Treatment Affect My Teeth?

During chemotherapy and radiotherapy, the saliva in your mouth, which usually acts as a protection against bacteria, dries up. This is why you may have a dry mouth, sore gums and changes in taste. Once the saliva dries up, many people start to drink more, and, in some cases, they will turn to sugary drinks. This, of course, is the worst thing you can do because sugar then attacks your mouth without the protection of saliva. It's not just sugar, though. Like other areas in your body, chemotherapy and radiotherapy can have an effect and teeth becoming loose or even falling out is the result. It can be avoided if you have any work needed before treatment starts so that your mouth is in the best condition possible, and you look after your oral health during treatment.

What Can I Do to Avoid Dental Problems?

As mentioned above, avoid sweet or sugary drinks. Even natural fruit juices fall into this category, but if your taste has changed so much that you're struggling to drink normally, please make sure you use sugar-free drinks.

Using a specialist toothpaste such as Duraphat (which can only be supplied on prescription) or Biotene (which is readily available) and investing in a soft-bristle brush will help. If you have an electric toothbrush, you can still use that but let the brush do the work – don't apply pressure. Duraphat will help with both fighting off bacteria and also lubricating your mouth, but you may want to invest in a mouth lubricant as well. Biotene has a good lubricant, but you must be careful that you're buying a lubricant rather than a mouthwash that may have alcohol and be quite painful.

If everything is very sore, then a mouthwash called Difflam is a good idea because it has a slight anaesthetic and takes the edge off any discomfort you may have.

Your GP and dentist will be able to prescribe these items and will also be able to tell you if there's anything better on the market.

I definitely had a very sore mouth during treatment but thankfully didn't suffer much beyond that (although one of my back teeth did crumble shortly after treatment stopped). Unfortunately, there are lots of cancer patients who have serious issues. The worst case I know of was a lady who had no problems before (although she didn't have her teeth checked before treatment) and lost nearly every tooth during and after chemotherapy. This is rare and extreme, but if you know there's a risk, it's better to do everything you can to prevent it from happening.

Accessing Dental Care and Dental Costs

This is where things get complicated. Across the UK, unless you're already registered with a dentist, it can be almost impossible to get an appointment and register as a new patient with a practice. If you are lucky and find a dentist taking on patients, it may only be for private care, and of course, that will have a knock-on effect on how much you need to pay for the work required.

In England, although cancer patients have free prescriptions after diagnosis, this doesn't apply to dental costs. Dental costs in Scotland, Wales and Northern Ireland also have to be paid for. I struggle to understand this because pregnant ladies get free dental care for 2 years. Cancer patients get nothing. This is fundamentally wrong, and I am currently campaigning the Government asking for this to change – with a focus on England in the first instance and hoping that the other nations will take on board any changes I manage to achieve. If you'd like to sign the petition, and it's free to do so, please visit this link:

https://www.change.org/p/free-dental-treatment-for-cancer-patients-change-the-law

In some areas of the UK, if you are on certain benefits, you may be able to reclaim costs, but these typically won't cover the full costs, and it's only those who don't work that can claim. For people who work and may not have any spare finances, there isn't any help, but you could approach cancer charities to see if there's an organisation in your area that might help.

In some parts of the country, there are dental hospitals (either attached to a hospital or standalone) – where treatment may be free, but some do charge depending on what needs to be done. Your GP and also your cancer team should be able to help.

It's becoming more common that an oncologist will want to see a dentist's clean bill of health before allowing you to have bisphosphonate treatment. Chemotherapy and radiotherapy normally will still go ahead, though.

CHAPTER 22

GENETIC TESTING

The Basics of Genetics and Breast Cancer

Prior to having cancer, I had very little knowledge of genetics other than maybe reading an article or seeing a TV programme. I suspect the majority diagnosed with breast cancer are in the same boat. As with everything, I've had to educate myself to find out what genetics mean for me and having breast cancer. I am far from an expert, but I've tried to write this chapter in an easy-to-understand way, but it's so confusing that I've struggled in parts not to boggle the mind! So, bear with me!

Like me, the only time you may have been aware of a defective gene relating to breast cancer is perhaps when a celebrity like Angelina Jolie speaks out about her brush with genetics. The most well-known genes that are a factor in increasing the risk of breast cancer are called BRCA1 and BRCA2. What exactly are the BRCA1 and BRCA2 genes? How do I know if I have them? What can I do about it? And what does it mean to my family and me?

Let's look first at how to pronounce BRCA and what it stands for. The pronunciation is "bracca", and the letters BRCA are made up of the words BReast and CAncer. It makes sense when you know that! But what are they, and what is a defective gene?

You may have read earlier (and forgive me if some of the information is repeated in this chapter) that we inherit 50% of our genes from our mother and 50% from our father. In some families, this means we also inherit genes that may have become "defective" – in other words, they have developed a manufacturing fault at some point in time that has become permanent and subsequently, they are passed down through our genes. We all have the BRCA genes, and if they haven't developed a fault (and the majority don't), they are not a risk factor for breast cancer, but when they are faulty, the risk of cancer can be as much as 80% higher.

Before we go any further, it's important to mention that the BRCA genes are not the only ones responsible for increasing our risk of breast cancer. There are actually many more, including PALB2, CHEK2, and ATM, to name a few. However, BRCA is the gene most commonly known.

How do you know if you have a defective gene? Typically, you won't be aware of it unless you have a family history of a specific type of cancer. With the BRCA gene, it could be breast, ovarian, prostate, or pancreatic cancer. However, as we discussed earlier in the book, our bodies can have a manufacturing blip at any point, causing genes to function incorrectly, so you may be the first in your family who has developed cancer. A defective gene can lay dormant and not have any impact at all, so you could go through life without cancer, but in others, the defective gene jumps into action, raises our risk, and we develop cancer.

The only way to know for sure if you're a carrier of a defective gene is to be tested. In England, there are NICE guidelines stating who should be tested, but, in my experience, in the UK, different hospitals use their own criteria. Private testing is available, and I'll link to that later, but for now, let's explore testing and what it may mean for you and your family.

Testing is very simple and just a blood test (or saliva if following the private route). However, before testing, it's normal that you meet with a geneticist who will assess your personal risk by asking questions about your family history of cancer (if any), your health, drugs/contraception you may have taken, age of first menstruation, age at menopause (if applicable) etc., to build a picture of the likelihood of risk.

If the geneticist believes there's a risk, they may suggest you go ahead with testing. However, it's at this point that you can decide whether to have it done or not. For some ladies, being told they are positive or negative can have a huge implication for their emotional state. For example, if you've tested and are negative, then you will still wonder, "why have I got breast cancer?" although there's a relief that you won't pass it on to your children. On the other hand, finding out you're positive for a defective gene can be a relief because you know why you've got breast cancer. This does mean that there are potential implications for your family, and it's quite common to feel very guilty. However, as I keep saying in this book, knowledge is power. If you have a defective gene, you can ensure your family is tested, that they have more screening at an earlier age, and/or they are given preventative surgery (as you may) if required.

Unfortunately, it can take months for the genetic testing to be analysed and for you to get the result. This may mean that you're already at the stage where you've had chemotherapy and surgery, so if positive for a defective gene, you may need to decide if you want to have further preventative surgery (perhaps a double mastectomy).

For obtaining a faster result, there's a company based in America that can privately analyse a saliva sample and normally get the result to you within a matter of weeks. The cost is around £300, and the test by this company is recognised (and used by) oncologists and geneticists in the UK. So, if you would prefer to go down that route, it may be speedier but a costly process. Also, unlike the UK test, which only tests for the BRCA and two or three other defective genes, the American company test for a much wider panel of genes. For more details, please read further on in this chapter.

Genetics in More Detail

It's important to note that having the BRCA1 or 2 genes only accounts for around 25% of ladies diagnosed with breast cancer (all types). So, what about the other 75%? Is it just bad luck that we've got breast cancer if we're BRCA negative? Let's have a look, more in-depth, at what a defective gene is and what we can do about it.

Genetics for breast cancer has progressed in leaps and bounds in the past few years, and with increased testing, more defective genes are being identified. The hope is that when specific corrupted genes are identified, it may be possible to analyse how and why they cause cancer and then potentially turn them off, thereby preventing cancer.

At a very basic level, it's necessary to explain that there are two distinct groups of defective or mutated genes.

The first type is called "germline", and these are the inherited genes like BRCA. As mentioned above, they're part of your DNA, and you can't change them.

So, this brings us to the second type of defective gene. If you think back to the very early chapters in this book, we looked at risk factors and how these can increase our risk of getting cancer. So, let's take "age" as a factor just as an example. As we age, our body can develop more defects as the cells divide and grow, and we are more susceptible to them copying incorrectly. This is when a genetic mutation can occur, and instead of being in our whole body, they may only be found in the tumour.

These mutations are called "somatic" or "acquired" mutations and are NOT part of your DNA and are NOT inherited. These are the ones that are typically responsible for our cancer and are the result of a manufacturing blip in our body. For breast cancer, one of these genes has the fantastic title of SMURF2, which makes me chuckle, although I appreciate it's not a laughing matter. Another that has been directly linked to breast cancer is TP53/p53, but of course, there are others.

There are literally tons of mutations, and if you want to be mind-boggled, you can find lists and lists of them online! I'm not a geneticist, so I can't tell you if specific mutations are germline (inherited) or somatic (acquired) but having a germline or somatic mutation could well be the reason why our Triple Negative Breast Cancer started. So even though 75% of ladies are BRCA Negative, they may be positive for a somatic mutation.

At the moment, knowing what mutation we have (or don't have), apart from the BRCA gene, doesn't actually lead to a specific treatment. It might help point your oncologist in a direction, though. Certainly, somatic mutations are not routinely tested for in the UK because there are no specific targeted treatments, although it is known that certain ones will respond better to a particular chemotherapy. If you think back to the Lehman et al. study, you will see they linked subtypes of Triple Negative to various genetic mutations, and these include both germline and somatic, so research is constantly looking at ways to improve treatments.

Where testing can help is that you may be able to minimise your risk (and that of your family) of a future breast cancer. As a link has been established for BRCA positive ladies with breast and ovarian cancer, surgeons are usually inclined to suggest a double mastectomy and sometimes removal of ovaries as a precaution against future cancer if BRCA positive. Other strong links to the PALB2 and CHEK2 genes may also indicate preventative surgery.

Despite all this research, if you're positive for a high-risk breast cancer gene, treatment is usually in the form of surgery rather than a wonder pill to prevent cancer from forming. However, there's some research that is pointing the way to developing a treatment similar to hormonal treatments that may well do this in the future.

As genetics is a fast-moving science, there are genes being identified all the time. Sometimes, a specific gene is identified, but the risk associated with it is unknown. In these instances, your result may show a gene listed as "VUS". This means a variant of uncertain significance. Typically, if you have one of these, your genetics team will keep your information on file, and as science progresses, if anything can be linked to your particular VUS, they may well get back in touch to discuss any new findings.

Just to throw another spanner into this already complicated arena, if you have two tumours, they may express different mutations! AND, if you test positive for the BRCA gene, your tumour may also have a somatic (acquired) genetic mutation. Therefore, finding a treatment that is a "one size fits all" is incredibly challenging.

In the meantime, just to show you how research is helping Triple Negative, here's an extract from a research paper. You may need to read it a couple of times for it to make sense, but I found it interesting (I'm an anorak)!

"........ Using a method that accounts for differences in tumour purity, we found a striking anti-correlation between

ER levels and the number of expressed mutations. That is, tumours with high levels of ER express fewer mutations than cancers with low ER. We formally modelled this relationship and determined that, for every 1% decrease in ER expression, 15 more mutations are expressed. As a breast cancer loses oestrogen receptor expression and becomes more transcriptionally active, it is more likely to actually express its complement of somatic mutations. For example, we found that TP53 mutations are more likely to be expressed in ER– than ER+ breast cancers. While speculative, this is of interest to researchers in the field of immunotherapy, since somatic mutations can act as neoantigens that trigger host immune responses......... "

So basically, in one of their studies, the authors looked at ER+ tumours - the more positive for oestrogen the tumours were, they discovered they were less likely to have mutations, so they were more "pure". The important bit for anybody with Triple Negative is that for each 1% decrease in oestrogen, 15 more mutations were found. So, by the time it gets to ER- (which all of us with Triple Negative are), there are lots more mutations, and they commonly found TP53 within those. As suggested in the last sentence, this might be of help in determining whether immunotherapy and/or other drugs will help us or not.

It's such a confusing area, but I hope this helps demystify genetics a bit. Wading through research papers when you're not medically trained is a bit like undertaking brain surgery with a knife and fork, but I hope the above gives you an insight into genetics!

What if My Health Authority Won't Test Me?

As I've mentioned above, you may want a full genetics screening, or your Health Authority may have refused to test you, and you may want to look elsewhere for help. If that's the case, there are companies that will specifically test for a much wider range of mutations but at a cost.

My genetics consultant, based in Manchester, recommended a company he uses called Color, which is based in America (www.color.com/product/overview). The current cost is approximately £300-350 for the "extended" kit (the one that's recommended), which includes postage and packaging to the UK. The cost may be different if the currency exchange rate changes, but this gives you an idea of the amount being charged in 2022.

The process is very simple. You order and pay for the kit online, and they send it to you in the post. This usually arrives within a week. You return a sample of saliva by post, and they will email (or mail) you the result in approximately 4-6 weeks. I know of ladies who have been emailed a result in a week, so it can be quicker. Currently, the mutations tested for are shown below, but this does change. Check their website for up-to-date information. Not all have been linked to breast cancer, but it's a broad genetic test:

BRCA1, BRCA2, MLH1, MSH2, MSH6, PMS2, EPCAM, APC, MUTYH, MITF, BAP1, CDKN2A, CDK4, TP53, PTE,

STK11, CDH1, BMPR1A, SMAD4, GREM1, POLD1, POLE, PALB2, CHEK2, ATM, NBN, BARD1, BRIP1, RAD51C AND RAD51D

CHAPTER 23

FERTILITY, PERIODS, MENOPAUSE, HRT, HORMONES

Preserving Fertility

If you are a younger lady, you'll have noticed that one of the questions in the section of things to ask your oncologist is about preserving fertility. If you are keen to have children in the future, it is important you discuss this with your oncologist at the first opportunity. Among other side effects to your fertility, chemotherapy can affect the number of eggs in your ovaries, and, apart from bringing on a temporary chemically induced menopause, it can also bring on menopause earlier.

There are various options that may be available, but (as with everything else), what you may be offered is individual for your circumstances. However, the following may be suggested:

- Ovarian stimulation to collect eggs for freezing.

- Freezing embryos – like the above, but the eggs are then fertilised before storing.

- You may also be offered tablets/an injection/an implant to help preserve your fertility.

- A newer technique and not widely available in the UK at the present time is to remove an ovary (or small pieces of an ovary), store and freeze them. This can be put back into your body after treatment has finished, which may help you to become pregnant naturally or with the help of IVF. The tissue removed contains many immature eggs that may give your fertility a boost once back in your body.

Periods

For all ladies who are pre-menopausal and still having periods, a side effect of having chemotherapy is that it throws women into chemically induced menopause. This means periods stop, your fertility is normally paused, and you can develop menopausal systems. For those already in menopause at diagnosis, there may be no change, but it can definitely heighten menopausal symptoms such as night sweats, hot flushes etc.

Whether you were pre or post-menopausal at diagnosis, unfortunately, this means that not only do you have the side effects from chemotherapy, but the menopause on top too!

It's impossible to predict how our bodies will react, but for pre-menopausal ladies, periods can stop immediately, or a few cycles in or, for a small number, not stop at all! If your periods have stopped, they typically return immediately fairly soon after treatment stops, but it could take up to two years for them to restart. If you were nearing menopausal age (typically late 40s, early 50s) but still having periods, your periods may not return, and you will continue into menopause. The body is a miraculous thing in that it concentrates on repairing "essential" parts of our body before it turns to things like hair, nails, fertility etc.

In normal circumstances (take cancer out of the mix), if you suspected you were peri-menopausal (i.e., the stage just before menopause), your GP could arrange for a blood test that would give an indication of whether you were peri-menopausal or not. The blood test is, however, only an indication because it can be unreliable. In order to be reasonably accurate, the test must be done on a set day of the month, between periods, and this is problematic if your periods are erratic, or you do not have them. So, their accuracy is debatable, but it may give you an indication.

For younger ladies, this unknown can be incredibly frustrating and worrying – especially if you haven't finished having a family. Just remember, it can take up to two years for everything to get back to normal.

Menopause / HRT / Hormones

What happens if you stay in menopause and are feeling rubbish – should you consider HRT? What are the risks?

A common misconception is that taking hormones is a "no no" ONLY for ladies with hormonal breast cancers. Wrong! Ladies with Triple Negative should NOT be taking hormones unless there's an overwhelming medical reason and the risks are fully understood.

I can hear you asking, but why? Triple Negative isn't fed by hormones! Correct. However, think back to an earlier chapter where we discussed how many breast cancers start off as hormonal and then lose their receptors as they grow and turn Triple Negative. That indicates that at some point, hormones may have played a part in our cancer.

Now think of something else .... If you have joined any online groups for breast cancer, you may have noticed how many pregnant ladies have been diagnosed with breast cancer? Some have had IVF, but the one thing they have in common is that their hormones will have changed. Does this start cancer? The medical professionals don't know for sure, but given the high number of young ladies, this happens to indicate to me that this is a high probability.

Also, the same can be said for menopausal ladies – again, they have a change in hormones in their bodies, and it can be around the same time they are diagnosed with breast cancer.

So, looking at all of the above – would you risk taking hormones?

Interestingly, despite the fact I tested negative for any genetic mutations, my daughter has been told by several different consultants that she should avoid taking any form of hormones. Whilst this may be super cautious, it does make me think the correlation is there.

If that doesn't convince you, I want to replicate below (and will include a link to the page) an analysis by researchers of 4 studies that involved over 4,000 women. The studies investigated ladies who had had breast cancer and looked at the correlation between cancer and HRT.

"About the study

This study was a meta-analysis, a study that combines and analyses the results of a number of earlier studies. In this case, the researchers analysed the results of four studies that included 4,045 women with a history of breast cancer.

Overall, 2,022 women were randomly assigned to receive HRT and 2,023 were randomly assigned to receive a placebo. The placebo was a pill that looked just like the HRT pill but contained no hormones. The women joined the studies about 2 years after they were diagnosed with breast cancer.

It's important to know that two of the four studies in the meta-analysis were stopped early because a short-term safety analysis found that using HRT increased the risk of breast cancer recurrence.

Overall, the researchers found that women who took HRT had a 46% higher risk of breast cancer recurrence versus women who didn't take HRT. This difference was statistically significant, which means that it was due to taking HRT and not just because of chance.

The researchers also looked to see if HRT's effect on recurrence risk was different for hormone-receptor-positive breast cancer and hormone-receptor-negative breast cancer.

Recurrence risk was:

- *80% higher in women diagnosed with the hormone-receptor-positive disease who took HRT*

- 19% higher in women diagnosed with the hormone-receptor-negative disease who took HRT

"We observed that the use of HRT is associated with a significant increase in the risk of recurrence among women with history of [breast cancer]," the researchers wrote. "Therefore, this approach remains contraindicated in the [breast cancer] setting. Future research should be focused on alternative safe interventions to mitigate menopause-related symptoms for these patients."

Written by: **Jamie DePolo**, senior editor

Reviewed by: **Brian Wojciechowski, M.D.**, medical adviser

The research was published online on Nov. 3, 2021, in the journal Breast Cancer Research and Treatment. Read the abstract of "Safety of systemic hormone replacement therapy in breast cancer survivors: a systematic review and meta-analysis."

Link = https://www.breastcancer.org/research-news/hrt-increases-recurrence-risk

So, to recap, the risk was so high that two of the four studies had to be stopped. That's incredibly frightening. This research suggests that the risk of having a recurrence for somebody who has previously had Triple Negative and taking HRT is 19% higher than for somebody who has had Triple Negative but doesn't take HRT. That's a very large percentage.

The majority of oncologists will tell you to avoid taking anything hormone-related – but a few will tell you that for

Triple Negative patients, it's safe to do so. You must do your own research and decide what's right for you.

I do understand that menopause can make your quality of life unbearable, but there are typically hormone-free alternatives, and I would urge you to explore these with your GP. In some parts of the country, there are menopause clinics that have specialists who may be able to help too.

In terms of practical things you can do to relieve menopause symptoms, there are quite a few avenues to explore, including acupuncture, and lifestyle changes, i.e., losing weight, keeping fit and exercising. There are also tablets, both prescription and herbal, that may help, including anti-depressants, blood pressure tablets, Oil of Evening Primrose and even a magnet that you wear 24 hours a day clipped to your underwear that has been proven in studies to help women with hot flushes (the LadyCare Magnet). I found this device purely by chance, and it worked amazingly well for me. I wore mine religiously, and my sleep became better, and my hot flushes lessened. However, there is a downside in that it's very easy to attach yourself to shopping trolleys which can be very amusing! Interestingly, NICE guidance does say to avoid the magnet if you've had breast cancer. I'm not sure why and there are actually hospitals in Scotland that give them to breast cancer patients, so I'm a bit confused as to who is right or wrong. At the end of the day, what works for one person may not work for another, but it's worth speaking to your GP and seeing what they can offer.

CHAPTER 24

YOUR LEGAL RIGHTS / FINANCIAL HELP

Employment Rights

This is a complicated chapter to write because laws are different in various parts of the UK, but the advice given below is reasonably generic. If you are in doubt, please get advice from a cancer charity such as Macmillan or Citizens Advice Bureau or take advantage of a free consultation with a solicitor.

In very broad terms, you are protected immediately at diagnosis for employment law purposes, and in easy-to-understand terms, it provides a halo around you so you can't be discriminated against for any reason <u>that relates to cancer</u>. The Legislation you are covered under at the time of writing is the Equality Act 2010 if you live in England, Scotland or Wales, or the Disability Discrimination Act 1995 (DDA) if you live in Northern Ireland.

There's no time limit to this protection, so even if you have finished all treatment and fully recovered, your employer cannot use your cancer to affect your employment. It also protects you if you apply for a new job.

Discrimination comes in many forms, some more obvious than others, but here are a few scenarios that would be considered discriminatory:

- Not allowing you to take time off work for medical appointments

- Demoting you (either financially or to a lesser demanding job because of your cancer)

- Not making reasonable adjustments/changes to your job – for example, if you have a manual role, allowing you to work in an office or environment where manual work can be eliminated or greatly reduced after surgery. Other examples may be refusing a request to work fewer hours to cope with fatigue etc. Reasonable adjustments must be related to your cancer, though.

- Giving you a warning or dismissing you due to the time you've had off sick or absences from work (if they're cancer-related).

- Dismissing you for any reason related to your cancer

- Suggesting you leave or retire

- Being difficult about paying you – including any sick pay you may be entitled to

- Allowing any form of harassment that can be related to your cancer or treatment, for example, laughing at your hair loss or criticising your work implying that you are "shirking" and not really ill

- Insisting on a return-to-work plan that you don't agree to and will feel unable to achieve.

- Changing your current job without consulting with you beforehand

- Employing somebody else to do your job on a permanent basis. However, advertising your role if it's temporary and will cease on your return is acceptable.

Some people choose to work through their treatment, and others need to take time off. This is very individual, but there are certain considerations, such as do you work in an environment where you may be more susceptible to infections – for example, a school or childminder? Do you work in a manual job where the work is very physical and demanding? Do you travel as part of your role and therefore won't be near to your team? This is not an exhaustive list, but I hope it prompts you to evaluate what's right for you.

Returning to Work After Treatment

There are no hard and fast rules that say you should return to work, for example, one month after all treatment has finished. It can take much longer for some to recover than others. You may have worked all through treatment, but whatever situation you are in, you do need to think about building back up to work slowly so that you're not exhausted. It's very important to allow your body to rest for it to repair. I do understand, though, that in some cases, finances will be an overriding factor and dictate what you do.

Some companies have an Occupational Health Department that can help with a return to work.

Occupational Health is normally a separate, outsourced part of the company and so independent. They will provide you and the company with advice based on medical evidence. Typically, they are the buffer between you and the company, and they will work with both sides to ensure a safe return to work.

A return to work is usually spread over a time period, gradually increasing each week until you're back to working your normal days and hours. A realistic timeframe is anywhere between 1 and 3 months, but it should be adjusted at any time if you're not coping well. A plan is agreed between you and your company based on what you think you may be able to work – this might be reduced hours and days or even a temporary change in role to reduce parts of your job that may cause you problems. If your role has been covered by somebody else in your absence, this might entail working alongside them and a handover. That can be tough but remember it's short term.

If your company doesn't have an Occupational Health team, then it may have a Human Resources Department or with small companies. It could be the management team or owner that you will discuss your return. A phased return to work is your right, so ask for this if you want it. Even if your company tells you you must return on the same hours and days as before, you don't have to. They are obliged to make "reasonable adjustments". Reasonable adjustments may be temporary OR permanent. The company cannot refuse to make changes unless there is a very good business reason why not. They would have to justify this at a Tribunal if legal action was taken against them.

However, there are certain circumstances where a company can terminate your employment if they can justify it's nothing to do with your cancer. For example, if the company is in financial trouble and must close a part of its business. If there are no other vacancies, and you are part of that business, they could legally make you redundant IF they are making everybody else redundant at the same time.

If they were reducing, say, 6 of the same job to 2, selecting you for redundancy would be problematic for them UNLESS they could justify that you were selected for reasons other than your cancer (so, for example, they would not be able to take your absence record into account). This can be really challenging for a company, and many times, they don't get it right, so if your job is under threat, it's worth seeking legal advice.

Don't forget; a company cannot suggest to a cancer patient that it may be easier to leave "in order to regain health". Whilst I'm sure in some cases that may be true, a company cannot and must not do this. If you have cancer, you have enough going on without feeling pushed into making a decision you don't want to. A company may offer an attractive financial package to end your employment, but unless this is something you really want, please don't accept it. In many cases, this is illegal and don't forget you'd be walking away from a pension, sick pay, holiday pay etc. as well.

Whilst thinking of a pension, if you're lucky enough to have a pension that allows retirement on the grounds of ill health, think very carefully about accessing it. Typically, there will be an age from which this is allowed, but you may lose money in the long term and have a lower pension. Please consider it very carefully and make sure you obtain independent financial advice.

The law is on your side. Try to think long term. Will you be able to get another job? When the money runs out, will you be able to cope? Get advice if you can because mentally, you may be feeling very weak and may just accept something for an easy life, especially if you're struggling with side effects.

Financial Help

It's a sad fact that most people diagnosed with cancer won't have prepared for an extended period off from work, and if you're self-employed, your entire income may be jeopardised.

Some companies will have a sick pay scheme that may be more generous than the statutory sick pay you get from the Government. Others will simply pay you statutory sick pay, and in some cases, they may not pay you at all, and you must claim sick pay directly from the Government. It can be a stressful time.

For help with financial matters, your local social security office or council, Citizens Advice Bureau (please ensure you visit the appropriate website for England, Scotland, Northern

Ireland or Wales) https://www.citizensadvice.org.uk/ and a government-backed website called Money Helper https://www.moneyhelper.org.uk/en can offer advice and assistance.

There are, however, at the time of writing, several state payment schemes designed to help you when you're unwell, and it's worth applying.

Employment Support Allowance

"Employment Support Allowance" or ESA has two sections, one that is means-tested (i.e., based on your income) and the other based on your National Insurance Contributions. The payments are split into two categories, a basic rate or enhanced rate, and your case will be assessed, and you may be awarded one or the other. ESA at the top rate (at the current time of writing is around £230 every fortnight, and if you normally work, the money you get will need to be taxed. This can cause all sorts of issues when you go back to work, so please make sure you speak with your payroll department and your local tax office because they will be able to adjust your tax code. ESA is normally assessed every year, but it can be ongoing if you continue to be ill.

Personal Independence Payment (PIP)

The other benefit is called "Personal Independence Payment", or PIP as it's also known. This is paid tax-free, and you can apply for it whether you work or not. It also has two rates of pay (basic and enhanced) and also two different parts, one for daily living and the other for mobility. To apply for PIP is, unfortunately, a lengthy and stressful process.

The first thing you have to do is complete a very long form that has about 30 questions! Each question has a set of criteria, and you have to detail how you are affected by cancer and treatments. Macmillan's can help you complete the form, and they always suggest you write it from the point of view of your worst day. You won't know how you'll feel or how you're affected until treatment starts, so it's difficult to submit the form until you get to that stage. After you submit the form, there is usually a 3-month wait (or longer) for an assessment. In most cases, you have a telephone (or face to face) meeting where an assessor will go through your answers. In a few cases, an assessment won't be needed if you've submitted lots of supporting evidence (i.e., letters from your consultants etc.).

After your assessment, you will receive a letter informing you of the decision, and if accepted, your payments will be backdated to the date you submitted your claim form. Your acceptance letter will also state when your PIP will be reviewed, and it is normally paid for 24 months before the review happens. If your cancer diagnosis is terminal, there is a form your GP can fill in, and your application is fast-tracked and unlikely to be reviewed.

To give you an indication of payments, if you were awarded both the daily living rate and mobility component at the basic rate, this would be approximately £84 per week.

The enhanced rate is around £154 per week. Unlike ESA, all PIP payments are tax-free.

If you are awarded the highest mobility rate, you may also be entitled to a Blue Badge from your local council, allowing you to park in areas set aside for disabled people. To apply, it is entirely separate and for information on how to do this, look at your local council's website.

Housing and Council Tax

If you are receiving benefits, depending on which, you may also be able to claim some, or all, of your housing or council tax costs. This is very individual because it depends on the benefit you're receiving, but if you visit your local council's website, there will be information on what is available.

Travelling Costs

Some hospitals will help with travelling costs to and from appointments. Your breast care nurse will know if there is such a scheme at your hospital. If there is, it's likely that you will be asked to provide proof such as a bus or train ticket etc.

Grants

Some charities will be able to help with a one-off payment to assist with increased heating bills, any adaptations that may be needed, travelling costs etc. Macmillan's offers a one-off grant of £350. Details can be found on their website (website information can be found in chapter 30).

Local authorities may also offer grants, but these differ from region to region. Please visit your local authority website or speak with your local councillor for more information.

Critical Illness Policies

You may have a critical illness policy (sometimes these are purchased at the same time when moving house), and if you do, it's worth claiming on that. Cancer is normally one diagnosis that is accepted without question, but, as with all insurances, there may be reasons why they won't accept your claim.

Travel Insurance

After a cancer diagnosis, getting travel insurance at a reasonable rate can be like pulling teeth! There are some companies that specialise in insuring cancer patients but check with your bank or credit card provider to see if they offer this as a "perk". If they do, please call them to ensure they will cover you. Normally they will, and it's just a quick phone call. If you're still undergoing treatment, they may not, but as soon as treatment ends, it might be easier. As a starting point, a list of companies that are generally kinder to cancer patients (in no particular order) are:

- InsureWith
- Avanti
- All Clear

- Insure & Go

- Get Going Insurance

- Insure Pink

- Colombus Direct

Be warned, though, that travelling as soon as treatment ends or even when you're undergoing treatment may result in an eye-watering quote.

In addition to the above, there is a government-backed website called Money Helper that has a directory of travel insurance companies for people with a pre-existing medical condition. https://www.moneyhelper.org.uk/en/everyday-money/insurance/travel-insurance-directory

You can also visit this website that compares travel insurance companies - again for those who have a pre-existing medical condition.

http://payingtoomuch.com/?fbclid=IwAR2HWBP7Jv5B2-4gP2RvlsFN9M4DkF_jM9Z-p-Fw6_S-w7TXrrYByGRlogQ

One thing I do want to mention, and I don't mean this to frighten or alarm anybody, is that it's quite common for ladies to want to book a holiday after treatment ends, and this is so, so tempting, especially after all you've been through, but please think this through very carefully. Our bodies take a while to heal, so going on a long-haul flight may result in blood clots. I don't say this lightly. Unfortunately, I know of a few people this has happened to. One lady, sadly, didn't take out travel insurance, had to pay for treatment abroad (scans etc.), but after flying home, died of a brain clot. This is incredibly sad and maybe could have been avoided. Short flights (under 3 hours) pose slightly less risk, but even then, the risk is there. A holiday in this country is much, much safer. Why not just wait 6 months for your body to be stronger? If you go away, the travel insurance will be higher than normal, but if things go wrong, you'll be glad you invested in it.

Medical Exemption Form

Don't forget, in England; you are eligible for free prescriptions the minute you are diagnosed. Your GP (or oncologist) will complete a form, and you will have to complete a section also. You then send it off, and quite quickly, you should be sent a medical exemption card. In Scotland, Wales, and Northern Ireland, prescriptions are free.

National Toilet Schemes

If you are undergoing chemotherapy or radiotherapy, it can change your bowel or bladder habits. There are two schemes that help you to access public toilets. The first is run by RADAR and is called The National Key Scheme (NKS). For a one-off fee of £4.75, you are provided with a key to access public disabled toilets. Should you wish to purchase one, contact Disability Rights UK via their website or call them on 0203 687 0790 (all information current at the time of writing but subject to future change).

The second scheme is run by Macmillan. It's called the Macmillan Toilet Card and consists of a free toilet card and keyring that you show to shop workers etc., whilst out in public, to explain that you may need to use their toilet facilities urgently. This is free, and details can be found on the Macmillan website (detailed in chapter 30).

CHAPTER 25

AFTER TREATMENT ENDS

You've finished treatment, and it's the day you have been waiting for! It's been a long time coming, but you're finally there, and it's all over, and you can put it behind you! Well, yes, that's what should happen in an ideal world, but in reality, you might feel a million miles away from the happy person you think you should be.

When you're having treatment, you're in a bubble knowing if you feel poorly or are worried, your team is there. Without knowing it, that gives you comfort, but as soon as treatment ends, that all stops. Not only that, but people will also expect you to be the "you" from before your cancer diagnosis. To them, you're "cured" and can get on with life. For some ladies, they may certainly feel that way, but for the majority, that's so far from the truth! Physically they may be right, but mentally it's a whole different ball game. If you were attacked by a lion and had tons of physical injuries, people could see that over time, you were healing, and they probably would understand how getting back to life would be difficult because they can imagine how tough it would be. Cancer, though, is different. They can't see it. The only thing they can equate cancer to is being ill, taking medicine, and then bingo, all back to normal.

For us, there's no bingo moment. Most of us will feel very different at the end of treatment. Coming to terms with having cancer is huge.

This is when the hard work starts, and your emotions can be totally out of control. You may feel alone, abandoned, and pressured into feeling happy that you've "beaten" cancer. Fears of recurrence may constantly plague you, and every ache or pain sends you into a tailspin. Does that sound familiar? If it does, it's because it's incredibly common. For some reason, nobody warns you what happens after treatment ends.

You may find this difficult to understand, but unbelievably, check-ups after treatment are normally only annual mammograms (or another scan if you have a mastectomy). For many ladies, that's a very, very long wait. People often ask why they're not offered scans more often, but some scans can give you low levels of radiation which is not what you want. There may be cost implications (not that you will think that's right), but lastly, frequent scanning can be really harmful to your mental health – although I appreciate not scanning enough, it does the same thing. So typically, you'll be told, "I'll see you in a year or if you have symptoms contact me sooner". I found that really daunting, especially as I had no symptoms in the first place!

Whilst I do believe it's helpful to have at least an ultrasound or mammogram every 6 months for 2 years after diagnosis, it's not usually possible for reasons of cost, the fact that scans are only as good as the day they're taken, and lastly, "scanxiety". That then leaves us with constant fear when we have an unexpected new ache or pain, wondering if it's back. Things we would have ignored before, suddenly, to us, maybe a sign of cancer. In reality, they very rarely are, but the thought is still there. I have a rule that I will give it two weeks to see if my new ache or pain resolves on its own and if it doesn't, I will see my GP. Normally, most things resolve in that two-week period.

Not only can it be difficult having to deal with your new normal, but how do you respond if somebody says, "so you're cured now". That used to stop me in my tracks. Yes, for now, I was free of cancer but was I cured? How do you respond? You don't want to say yes, but it's not right to say no. I told the truth that I'd been treated, and so far, so good, but my cancer has a high recurrence rate, so I've got to be vigilant. People seemed to understand that, but I'm not sure if they fully understood the impact.

The reality of life after chemo is tough for many of us. In fact, beyond tough. We have a new normal. A different normal and adjusting to that so that we can live again is the hardest part. It took me 18 months to get help, but when I did, I realised just how much I needed it.

There are other things we may have to deal with are the side effects of our treatment, which can be difficult to overcome.

Aches, Pains, Tiredness and Cognitive Issues

I really don't understand why cancer teams don't warn about how you might physically and mentally feel after treatment finishes (perhaps they're unaware), but in the Triple Negative Facebook group I belong to, one of the most common threads I see is "I've finished treatment and now feel like a 90-year-old", "I'm aching all over, is this normal?" "I can't remember simple names, and my brain feels like it's mud", and "why do I feel worse and have trouble walking after treatment when I should be feeling better"? Insert here any form of ache or pain!

Well, this is unfortunately very normal. Let's look at cognitive issues first. You might suddenly find you can't remember names. Mid-sentence, you may be talking and then lose the thread of what you were saying. You may look at a family member and can't even remember their name! It can be so bad that you may start to wonder if perhaps something more sinister is happening to you. It's not. This is what is glibly referred to as Chemo Brain and can be similar to Baby Brain (if you've ever been pregnant, this may have happened to you then). Although in my experience, chemo brain is ten times worse! I've always prided myself on my intellect and love watching quiz shows etc. Suddenly my brain felt as if I was wandering around in quicksand, and it was taking so long just to remember a simple answer. Does any of this sound familiar? Have a read of the section further in this chapter, where there are links to articles about cognitive issues. But for now, let's look at the new aches, pains, lumps and bumps.

Lumps and bumps that you haven't noticed before may suddenly be there and in the front of your mind – surgery may be the culprit here. Or it may be a pain in your rib area where radiotherapy might be the cause. Don't forget, as mentioned in the chapter on chemotherapy, surgery and radiotherapy, changes can occur for a year or two after treatment has finished, and for some reason, rib pain is the most common side effect to start later.

Peripheral neuropathy (i.e., tingling and numbness normally in hands and feet, although it can creep up arms and legs) can also get worse after treatment. This is normally a short-term side effect, but it can be dangerous because you may drop things or burn yourself. If this happens to you, please see your oncologist or GP. Certain medications can help, but you might be referred to a specialist who can investigate further.

These don't start the day treatment finishes. For many, they can start around 4-6 weeks after chemotherapy or radiotherapy ends (obviously, the timeline differs from person to person). You may wake up one day and feel like you're aching, either in just your legs, or your arms or simply everywhere. Just getting out of bed may really hurt. A stiff, heavy feeling and a sort of "I've been run over by a truck" feeling. If you've been sitting down for a while, you may experience this when you try to get up. You may feel like you've seized up and need to inch yourself gently into a standing position. For me, I had pain from my feet to my hips, and it was totally unexpected as, during chemotherapy, I hadn't suffered from this at all!

Tiredness (and sometimes breathlessness) are also side effects that take a while to resolve. If you need to have a nap, if you can, it's good to do so because it's your body signalling that it needs a bit of time to repair itself.

All this is incredibly worrying, and your first thought will be that cancer's back. Well, the "good" news, if you can call it that, is that most of these side effects are temporary. They are simply a late onset of side effects from chemotherapy, surgery and/or radiotherapy.

It's impossible to know when these issues will subside, but normally it's within six to twelve months, but certain side effects may take even longer to resolve.

Cancer Related Cognitive Dysfunction (Chemo Brain)

In terms of cognitive issues, this is one of the things that hit me hard. I'd be talking to somebody and completely lose my train of thought, or I'd use the wrong words. I honestly thought I had early-onset dementia, and it was so bad that it caused me considerable anxiety. When I found out this was normal and usually a temporary side effect, it did help me not to worry about it so much, but it didn't help with the frustration or embarrassment. I found that doing lots of crosswords and puzzles, whilst deeply exasperating, did help. Reading was also helpful, but my concentration levels were very short.

If you are working, and especially if you have a job where you need to be on the ball, having cognitive issues can be really distressing because you feel helpless. I know of a lady who is a solicitor, where her work depends on her memory and ability to analyse complex situations. She suffered really badly, and so did her work. The more she worried about it, the worse it got. It also didn't help that her employer just didn't understand how a once competent woman was struggling. This is really common, and it's not something that's easily explained – and can be embarrassing. I have found a few articles online that I will link to below because sometimes just having an article that you can print out and show somebody may help and also can make you feel less of a fraud (not that you are, but you may be worried that's how others see you).

Please remember, most of these side effects are short term and WILL resolve. Give yourself time to recover. Don't try to be the superhuman you were before the diagnosis. I apologise that the links are so long!

A link to an article about muscle aches:

https://www.cancer.net/coping-with-cancer/physical-emotional-and-social-effects-cancer/managing-physical-side-effects/muscle-aches?fbclid=IwAR2vaufL74T7F8v5pBlrD4Y_fuHjhDSTIfrja e5ha71Im74EC4FRJY8KzoQ

Links related to cancer-related cognitive dysfunction (i.e., chemo brain):

https://www.cancer.net/coping-with-cancer/physical-emotional-and-social-effects-cancer/managing-physical-side-effects/attention-thinking-and-memory-problems

https://www.macmillan.org.uk/cancer-information-and-support/impacts-of-cancer/chemo-brain

https://breastcancernow.org/information-support/facing-breast-cancer/going-through-breast-cancer-treatment/side-effects/side-effects-chemotherapy/cognitive-impairment-chemo-brain

https://owise.uk/what-is-chemobrain/?fbclid=IwAR3fZ_EQIAcEER1tzITfdGbkKpD8y0EBHdsSX44CCH1UAdmKB9lRSvZwj8g

Anti-Depressant Tablets

I have mentioned earlier that it's very common for ladies to need a little help at points, perhaps during and after cancer. Your GP will be able to prescribe anti-depressants if you feel they may help. They do take at least two weeks to kick in, so it's not an immediate fix, but when they start working, they should take the edge off your anxieties and worries and allow you to cope a little better. Just like with chemotherapy, one size doesn't fit all, so the dose and medication may need tweaking at points, but speak with your GP, who can help with this. It's absolutely no shame to take these tablets – you've been through an appalling time, and sometimes are minds just need the pressure taken off them.

Counselling

You may never have considered that you need counselling or help with depression and anxiety, but when treatment concludes, you may suffer from a form of Post-Traumatic Stress Disorder. I definitely did. You may suddenly have feelings of being overwhelmed. You may cry for no reason, be in a bad mood that you can't shift, snap at people around you and generally find it difficult to move forward. You may even feel jealous that people around you are happy when you feel you're dying inside. Does any of that sound familiar? I described to my counsellor that I felt like a leaf that was curling up around the edges and dying.

Talking, especially with a counsellor who specialises in cancer, can be incredibly beneficial because how you're feeling will be very familiar to them, and they will reassure you that you are certainly not going mad, and your feelings are normal. You've been through one of the most traumatic events you will ever experience in your lifetime. Your health and the way you view it may have changed. Your appearance may have changed. You may feel that you don't want to plan anything just in case you're ill again. You may see other cancer patients moving on with their lives, and it can give you unrealistic expectations that you're not recovering as fast as you should.

One thing I learned from my own counselling was that I shouldn't compare myself to anybody. My counsellor said to me, "do you realise you keep saying you "should" be feeling happier – who says you "should"? And she was right. I was putting way too much pressure on myself.

One thing that happened, and I'm sharing it with you because it may happen to you, is that I met a lady in one of the Triple Negative groups who was diagnosed one month before me. We were friends on Facebook, and when our treatment ended, I noticed she was posting so many "positive" posts about moving on, exciting things she had planned, things she was doing etc. I used to look at those posts, and it made me feel useless like I was failing in my recovery.

After about 6 months of seeing those posts, I mentioned it to my counsellor. She said, "You never know what's really going on in someone's life – they will only post what they want you to see," and I thought about it and realised that might be the case, but I wasn't wholly convinced. Just by chance, a few weeks later (as if she could see inside my head), my friend posted again, but this time it was to say, don't be fooled by my upbeat posts. The reality is that I'm struggling to cope and move forward and picking up the pieces is really difficult. Seeing that, and talking with my counsellor, really helped, and I suddenly gave myself permission to recover at my own pace. You must do that too.

Please reach out and get help if you need it. There are lots of cancer charities that may help, but even speaking to others in online Facebook groups will help because they're in the same position and will understand without judgement. Get help wherever you can, for as long as you need it.

CHAPTER 26

FUTURE DEVELOPMENTS - TRIPLE NEGATIVE BREAST CANCER

Since I was diagnosed in 2016, although the main treatment has remained almost the same for Triple Negative, there have been changes such as adding in Carboplatin, Capecitabine (and very soon, hopefully, immunotherapy for early breast cancers). So, there have been advances.

Drug Trials

The amount of research into developing new drugs for Triple Negative is vast and spans the globe. It's actually a very challenging area for researchers and so can be an interesting subject, so there are always trials happening, specifically for Triple Negative Breast Cancer.

Trials are designed differently according to the drug, but they all have an entry criterion that must be met before being accepted. There are usually a limited number of places available on each trial. Some are large, into the thousands, but others are much smaller, with under 50 participants. Trials are conducted at some hospitals around the UK (different trials use different hospitals), so you may be lucky, and there's one near you. Alternatively, you may want to travel to a nearby hospital. To be put forward for a trial, your oncologist must submit your details to the trial team (you can't do it yourself).

Trials are grouped into phases 1, 2 and 3. A phase 1 trial is the first time that the drug will be tried on a human, and usually, these are smaller trials, but their safety will have been tested, as far as possible, to eliminate potential issues before getting to phase 1. Phase 2 will follow a phase 1 trial if phase 1 has proved to have promise. Phase 3 is usually the last phase and will be a bigger trial. Results from this trial will normally determine whether the drug goes to market or will be licenced for the use that the drug manufacturer has designed it for.

Some trials guarantee a set of treatments, but others have different sections where some patients receive a placebo, and the other set would receive the trial drugs. This is, of course, to determine if the drugs are really effective, but typically, for early breast cancer, there is some form of the drug. Some trials have more than two sections with different drug combinations, and you may or may not know which group you'll be in. Your oncologist is unlikely to know either. One thing's for sure is that you won't be left without treatment, but there is a risk (albeit small) that the new drug may not suit you – but that's the same with all drugs, even with the chemotherapies that we are given as standard.

Drug trials are, of course, essential to developing more tools to defeat cancer. However, the way trials are designed means you may never know if you've been given the new drug or not. Not all trials substitute what you would normally have in terms of a treatment regime.

Some trials are designed after the main treatment has ended to determine whether there are ways to detect a potential recurrence. These trials can be reassuring as you're being constantly monitored, BUT this can also be stress-inducing. Having constant tests and perhaps not being informed about the results (which can happen on trial) can be quite tough to mentally cope with. So, before you decide to join a trial, please think about how this may affect you. It's not good for the trial if you start but then stop a short way into it, so have a think about whether a trial is a right route for you.

If you want to see a list of current "open" trials, they can be found online at https://www.cancerresearchuk.org/about-cancer/find-a-clinical-trial, and by typing Triple Negative into the search bar, it will bring up specific trials that are open. However, each trial has its own eligibility criteria, so please read the appropriate section.

Identifying Cancer Cells Before They Show on Scans (ctDNA)

Between 2017 to 2019, a trial called c-TRAK was launched in the UK. Its purpose was to use blood from patients who had previously had breast cancer to see if they could identify cancer cells before they could be detected by a scan. This looked at something called circulating tumour DNA or ctDNA. Researchers know that when breast cancer cells die, they can release small pieces of DNA into the bloodstream, and this is what is referred to as circulating tumour DNA (ctDNA). So, doctors have developed a new test that looks for ctDNA in the blood.

The presence of ctDNA might indicate that the patient may have a recurrence or potentially metastatic cancer. This is a very exciting advancement because if it can accurately identify patients at risk, there's a possibility of giving treatment early to remove the risk. The trial is now closed, but this is a "watch this space" moment. Results from the trial are expected at some point in 2022, and if positive, it could mean there's a test for early detection and then earlier treatment of breast cancer!

Zest Trial – ctDNA Monitoring/Parp Inhibitor Treatment

Following the c-TRAK trial, a new Phase 3 trial was launched in 2021 to study 800 patients who have had Triple Negative breast cancer. This trial monitors those on the trials using ctDNA, but in addition, half the patients will receive a drug called Niraparib (a PARP Inhibitor – please see below for further information) and the other half a placebo.

Patients will be regularly tested using "Signatera", which is a custom-built circulating tumour DNA (ctDNA) test for treatment monitoring and molecular residual disease (MRD) assessment in patients previously diagnosed with cancer. The Signatera test is personalised and tumour-informed, providing each individual with a customised blood test tailored to fit the unique signature of clonal mutations found in that individual's tumour. This maximises Signatera's accuracy for detecting the presence, or absence of, residual disease in a blood sample, even at levels down to a single tumour molecule in a tube of blood. Signatera is intended to detect and quantify how much cancer is left in the body, detect recurrence earlier, and help optimise treatment decisions. Based on these results, the trial team will be able to determine whether taking Niraparib will prevent a recurrence or not. If this trial is successful and patients taking Niraparib have a lower or reduced rate of recurrence, this may be an exciting way forward for Triple Negative breast cancer patients.

PARP Inhibitors

PARP Inhibitors are a relatively new drug, and in 2016, when I was diagnosed, they were being trialled in patients who carried a genetic mutation such as BRCA 1 and 2. As you've read earlier, the body attempts to repair both healthy and cancerous DNA, and if a patient carries a specific genetic mutation, PARPS can be used to do this. BRCA patients lack a specific pathway that repairs a certain part of the DNA which means they're more susceptible to a strike by cancer. If a patient with a genetic mutation is treated with a PARP inhibitor such as Olaparib (also known as Lynparza) or Talazoparib, the cancers are no longer able to multiply, and they die.

Both drugs have already been licenced in the UK to treat patients with metastatic breast cancer who have a defective gene, and studies have shown that they have the ability to slow down cancer, improve the quality of life and prolong life expectancy.

Further studies have shown that giving PARP Inhibitors to patients with early (primary) breast cancer who have the BRCA gene can reduce recurrences.

The downside is that this may only be for BRCA positive patients, and also, these drugs can have side effects. However, it's a step in the right direction, and it's expected that they will be licenced in the UK for use at some point in 2022. Interestingly, the Zest trial mentioned above is being trialled on patients with both BRCA positive and negative status, which will be interesting to see how negative patients react,

Immunotherapy:

Immunotherapy drugs are now more accessible, and in the next few years, I'm sure there will be more options available for primary breast cancer. Hopefully, with the possible licencing of Pembrolizumab, this may open the door for other trials and licencing. The good news is that new immunotherapy drugs are being tested all the time, so this is an area that's growing.

Trodelvy (Sacitzumab Govitecan) – Antibody Drug Conjugates

One of the most exciting drugs to have been developed is a drug called Trodelvy, inherited and now made by Gilead. Very simply, "antibody-drug conjugates" work by identifying cancer as a target and then work with a specific drug (in this instance, Trodelvy) to home in on that target. With Trodelvy, a target called TROP2 has been identified, and this is found in about 90% of all Triple Negative cancers. Given that Trodelvy has a specific target, the thinking is that it's more likely to find cancer and destroy it. Certainly, in trials in America, there were some really astonishing results with stage 4 breast cancers, especially in patients who had previously had two different types of chemotherapy that had failed. Trodelvy has been used in America now for a few years, and it does seem to be one drug that has better than average results.

Of course, there will be patients for whom it won't work and some who will be on it long-term, and it may stop working (but that's the same for all drugs). It also does have some harsh side effects, and hair loss is a given with this treatment.

As at April 2022, Trodelvy has been approved for use in the UK, but funding has not yet been agreed in England, Wales or Ireland. This is incredibly disappointing because it means it's not available for patients. Encouragingly, Scotland have agreed funding and Trodelvy is available to patients in that part of the UK.

Breast Cancer Now and other charities are lobbying hard for NICE to agree funding and hopefully, NICE and Gilead will come to an agreement. If/when they do, it should be available to patients throughout the UK.

In the meantime, up until NICE refused funding, the manufacturer, Gilead, allowed UK stage 4 patients access to the drug on compassionate grounds. So, there are already UK patients receiving Trodelvy, with the first patient being treated in December 2021.

The exciting news is that in America, Trodelvy is now also used for early breast cancers as well (ie stages 1-3). Although it's too early to evaluate what impact it may be having, typically, the UK follows America, so trials may well start soon. This is definitely promising news for defeating Triple Negative and certainly one to watch.

CHAPTER 27

NATURAL / ALTERNATIVE OR COMPLEMENTARY REGIMES

LifeMel Honey to Help with Low Neutrophils

I am very reluctant to promote a product, but there is one that I know can help around 90% of cancer patients to keep neutrophils within the desired level and avoid treatment delays.

I first became aware of this product, which is honey, by watching This Morning and a segment with Dr Chris Steele, their resident doctor. He explained that he tells his patients to take LifeMel honey to keep their neutrophil levels in the range required for chemotherapy to go ahead, and in most cases, it works.

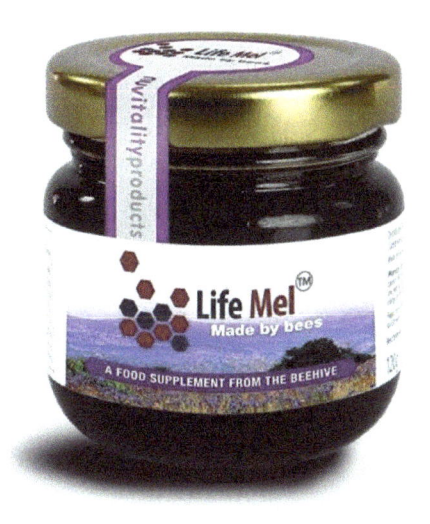

It's a particular honey that's made in Israel, and the unique properties stem from the food that feeds the bees. I was very sceptical, but over the years, I've seen it help a huge percentage of ladies undergoing chemotherapy. I have to be very clear that there is NO evidence base that this honey works, and the only reason I am suggesting trying it is that I have anecdotal evidence from hundreds of Triple Negative cancer patients. The other reason I am more comfortable suggesting this product is that you may well have honey on your toast in the morning for breakfast or on your porridge! Honey is normally safe to take (unless you're diabetic or have another medical condition that prevents you from doing so), so if you're in doubt about taking this, you MUST speak with your oncologist.

The honey is produced by a company called NuVitality and is called LifeMel and is in a tiny 120g jar, which unfortunately is costly. One jar will only last about 3 weeks, and at around £40, it can be expensive, BUT if it keeps you out of the hospital, avoids chemotherapy delays and keeps your neutrophils high, then you may think it's worth every penny. You have to take one level teaspoon under the tongue in the morning and the same again at night. You take this every day (not just for a few days). The honey has a very distinct taste – some people love it, and others hate it! I guess the way to look at it is that the majority of things that make you better don't taste nice!

I know of ladies who have become quite ill with low neutrophils and have had their chemotherapy cancelled, and who decided to try the honey. In the majority of cases, they've been astounded to find it works, and their neutrophil levels have been in the acceptable range for the next chemotherapy – so no more delays. One lady, after taking this for a few cycles, thought she'd been cured, so she stopped taking the honey and ended up back in the hospital with low neutrophils! Needless to say, she went straight back onto it and didn't have any further issues.

If you want to try the honey, it can be purchased from Amazon, but please make sure you take it as directed and take it every day. NuVitality does make a number of different kinds of honey, but this is the one you want. If your neutrophils are doing well, you may want to try just one teaspoon a day, and that may be sufficient for you. Please note, I am not affiliated with this company in any way, nor am I being paid to promote this product and, as mentioned above, there is no trial or evidence to suggest it either works or doesn't.

Diet

As I've said in an earlier chapter, there are so many myths about changing your diet, such as drinking lemon in hot water, drinking milk infused with turmeric, cutting out sugar, detoxing using various methods, changing to being a Vegan etc., and if these things make you feel better and it's something you want to do in general, then it will be the right thing for you. However, please do not think that anything you have eaten has caused your cancer.

Cancer Research UK has a page on their website debunking food/drink myths relating to cancer (https://www.cancerresearchuk.org/about-cancer/causes-of-cancer/diet-and-cancer/food-controversies). In a nutshell, they conclude that none of the following cause or prevent cancer:

- Sugar
- Artificial sweeteners
- Eating burnt food
- Eating tomatoes (tinned or fresh)
- Green Tea does not prevent cancer
- Soy products do not affect cancer risk

Macmillan has similar information:

(https://www.macmillan.org.uk/cancer-information-and-support/impacts-of-cancer/healthy-eating-and-cancer/common-questions-about-diet-and-cancer)

The BDA – Association of UK Dieticians - has a myth-busting page about food and cancer that can be found online at https://www.bda.uk.com/resource/challenging-cancer-diets-myths.html. They, too, have a table on their website that states the following do not cause cancer:

- Dairy
- Soya
- Alkaline
- Sugar
- And they give a warning about taking supplements when undergoing treatment.

I can't stress enough that a healthy diet with a bit of what you fancy is far more likely to make you feel happier! After my treatment ended, I asked my oncologist if I should follow any particular dietary advice, and he recommended a Mediterranean style diet, basically having lots of vegetables, lean meat, and olive oil. It doesn't stop cancer, but it's a good way to ensure you're getting nutrients.

Alternative/Complementary Regimes

There is a growing (and alarming trend) on the internet and, in particular, social media platforms promoting ways of beating and starving cancer. I won't name them, but it's usually an individual (with no or little medical background) who has done some research, been treated and is now cancer-free. What they may not tell you is that their cancer was discovered early. It might have been a non-aggressive type. They had conventional treatment but then took their own "cure" as well. In some instances, you have to pay money to join a group or buy products.

There are also clinics all over the world promoting curing cancer. They are very convincing and usually run by oncologists or teams of doctors. Again, I can't stress this enough – THERE IS NO CURE FOR TRIPLE NEGATIVE CANCER AT THE PRESENT TIME! Sometimes these clinics will run complementary therapies alongside traditional ones (such as oxygen therapy, dendritic cell therapy, vitamin infusions), but none of these clinics can actually cure cancer. Whilst I could tell you horror stories of people I've known who have fund-raised over 6 figures to pay for treatment abroad, ultimately, they have spent time away from their loved ones and undergone treatment that has been no more successful than they could have had at home.

Lastly, I would like to mention alternative cures such as the alkaline diet etc. Whilst there may be some limited truth in all the alternative cures you may come across, the reality is that Triple Negative Breast Cancer, if left to its own devices, won't be kind to you.

When I was first diagnosed, I came across a series of videos uploaded to YouTube by Christina Newman. She was very much anti-chemotherapy and put her faith in alternatives. She tried many, many different methods, but ultimately, after documenting the lack of results, she turned to traditional treatments. Although her story doesn't have a happy outcome, the traditional treatments allowed her to live quite a few years after diagnosis and go on to have a beautiful baby daughter. Her videos are a sombre reminder that chemotherapy can be your friend. A link to her videos:

https://www.youtube.com/channel/UCtwtZPP3Q1M2uuQwkeTHNgw

Repurposed Drugs

Lastly, there is a growing trend in the UK to take repurposed drugs (i.e., drugs that are licenced and used to treat medical conditions other than cancer). For example, metformin is used in the management of diabetes. The thinking is that these drugs block "pathways" in the body to prevent cancer from forming. Typically, patients are advised to take a cocktail of around 10-20 repurposed medicines and herbal remedies, which patients pay for via private clinics.

Whilst some of these drugs may help, my concern is that at the time of writing, there are no long-term clinical trials and no published data that include a large group who either have or have had cancer, compared to placebos. Some of these clinics publish their own small-scale data, but in order for a trial to truly be a trial, trial conditions together with a good reference sample of people need to be included.

Some patients will take these drugs without telling their oncologists. Some will tell their oncologists. My view, and it's only my view, is that taking drugs long term that is NOT proven to prevent cancer can lead to other complications. If you decide to investigate further, please make sure you ask your oncologist for his/her advice and do a lot of research (not just reading one book) to determine if this is something you want to do. Analyse what you're being told objectively. If somebody says they're cured, look at their diagnosis, their treatment etc. Quite often, what you're told is not the full picture.

CHAPTER 28

THINGS I WISH I'D KNOWN AT DIAGNOSIS

All the information below is elsewhere in the book, but I thought it might be useful to just make a list, with the benefit of hindsight!

1. Between diagnosis and treatment, starting emotionally is very difficult.
2. Do not Google
3. Join online specialist Triple Negative groups.
4. Know that once treatment starts, you may begin to feel calmer.
5. You haven't done anything to start your cancer.
6. Tumour size doesn't matter!
7. Get your teeth checked before treatment starts.
8. Have your eyebrows microbladed before treatment starts (if you want)
9. LifeMel honey to keep your neutrophils healthy. If it doesn't work – stop!
10. Do NOT worry if you have surgery and then chemotherapy or the other way around.
11. If offered a central line – a PICC or Port, have it
12. Chemotherapy is your friend – not your enemy.

13. Chemotherapy is a MUST.

14. Chemotherapy is "doable".

15. Don't take your worldly possessions in a suitcase to your chemotherapy appointments!

16. Steroids - do not take them too late; otherwise, you'll be awake all night!

17. If you are suffering from nausea or any side effect, reach out to your team.

18. Expect to have treatment delays.

19. Hair loss starts around days 17-23. Brows and eyelashes will be the last to depart.

20. Seek help. Never suffer in silence. This is relevant at any point in your treatment or after.

21. Aches, pains, and cognitive issues are common after treatment. They start around 4-6 weeks after treatment ends. This is NORMAL.

Remember - YOU CAN DO THIS

CHAPTER 29

SURVIVOR STORIES

Just as I was finishing writing this book, I decided to ask people in an online group what they would like to read if they bought a book about Triple Negative. Thankfully, I had covered most of the subjects mentioned, but Annabel, who was treated for Triple Negative over 20 years ago and remains cancer-free, suggested having a section with "real life" survivor stories. An excellent idea, and there's no better way to end this book!

The following are stories, written in their own words, by ladies who are 10 years and more beyond diagnosis who were diagnosed with Triple Negative Breast Cancer. Their stories are overwhelmingly inspiring and, I'm sure, will give you hope and strength. Let's start with Annabel's journey!

Annabel's Story – Diagnosed 2002

I'm Annabel Chown, and I was a 31-year-old single architect from London when I was diagnosed with Triple Negative breast cancer in 2002.

I felt a lump in my left breast in the early hours of a Sunday morning while getting ready for bed after a party. As soon as I felt it, I panicked that it was cancer, even though (at the time) there was no history of breast cancer in my family. My GP reassured me it felt benign, but he sent me for an ultrasound. The ultrasound indicated a benign lump, but as the needle biopsy showed some slightly unusual cells, the surgeon decided to remove it 'as a precaution.'

His last words to me before I was taken down to the operating theatre were, 'Don't worry, it's definitely not cancer.' But I came to from the anaesthetic, only to be told that it was, after all, cancer.

At that moment, my world fell away. Suddenly I was being sent off for scans to check if cancer had spread and told I needed to see an oncologist. Luckily, it hadn't spread, my lymph nodes were clear, and my tumour was a small one, at 12mm. But because it was an aggressive Grade 3, Triple Negative and because I was so young, the oncologist told me I would definitely need chemotherapy, as well as radiotherapy. He also told me, in one breath, that my hair would probably fall out, and I might be left infertile by the treatment.

I was prescribed 6 cycles of FEC chemotherapy and 30 sessions of radiotherapy, which was the standard treatment back in 2002. Chemo made me feel very sick, and I did indeed lose almost all my hair, despite wearing an ice cap. It didn't make me infertile, though, and my periods came back after.

Completing treatment was a surprisingly hard time for me. I thought I'd feel great once it was over, but I actually felt terrified and quite low, being back in the so-called real world and away from what had become the security of the oncology unit and its treatments. Plus, it was only then that the magnitude of what I'd been through really hit me, especially as it felt like all my friends had spent the past year just getting on with their lives, dating, marrying, moving ahead with their careers – the kinds of things you're meant to be doing in your early 30s.

But after about six months, I started to feel more like myself again, and I decided that I was going to use the experience as a catalyst to create some positive changes in my life. So, I decided not to return to my high-pressure job in an architect's practice and instead set up as a freelance architect, working from home. Cancer taught me that life could be short, and I wanted to make sure I now had time for all the things in my life I loved, such as yoga, writing, and my friendships.

A few years later, I also trained to become a yoga teacher, which is what I mostly do now. I eventually signed up for online dating, too, which is where, in 2010, I met my now-husband. Around that time, life threw me another surprise, though: two of my cousins were, in close succession, diagnosed with breast cancer, and it turned out that my family carries the BRCA1 mutation. I've since had a risk-reducing mastectomy, and (after I had my son) I had my ovaries removed.

I thought my life was over the day I heard those awful words, 'You have cancer.' It's hard to believe that almost 20 years have now passed, and here I am with the husband and child I feared I might never have.

Julie's Story – Diagnosed 2009

My name is Julie Morris, and I live in Leicester. I was diagnosed in 2009 with Triple Negative breast cancer at age 43. I found the lump by self-examination because 6 years earlier, my sister, at the age of 40, had been diagnosed with Triple Negative breast cancer, so I was more aware of checking myself.

My tumour was 2.4cm, and I also had 3 lymph nodes involved. At the time, I thought I was bound to die because my sister had survived, and so I didn't think the odds were in my favour and I would be the one. I had 6 FEC-T chemotherapies, and during my first and second chemo, I was so sick I thought my stomach would turn inside out. By the third, I think my body had got used to it! The next 3 were taxol which had different side effects, including no sense of taste, which at the time was horrible. I've had covid recently, so I was used to having no sense of taste!

When I was first diagnosed, it seemed like the end, but my sister helped and said my wall was right in front of me, and the further I got away from the diagnosis, the more the wall would move into the distance just like hers. I held on to that, and now I can hardly see the wall at all.

With my sister and me both having Triple Negative, we agreed to be genetically tested, which, I won't lie, was quite stressful. We went for the results, and after they told my sister she didn't have BRCA1 or 2, I was happy for her but was, in bits, thinking I must have the gene. I had to wait a further week until they rang me and amazingly, I didn't carry them either! However, we were asked if they could keep our information on file and test for other genes that may be discovered in the future – both my sister and I agreed.

I am now 13 years on, my sister is 19, and life is good. Yes, I do still worry if I get a pain I haven't had before, and I still check myself regularly. My nails don't grow, and one boob is smaller than the other, but I'm here, and I'm so grateful every day.

Marian's Story – Diagnosed 2010

Marian Catt - I was 49 in 2010 with two grown-up daughters. I had been going along happily with my everyday life then; I found a lump, and life changed overnight. I used to check my breasts in the shower regularly. On 12 December 2010, whilst sitting with a glass of wine, my hand brushed my left breast, and I felt a lump. Up to that point, I wasn't aware of its existence at all. I was very quiet and took myself to bed and cried. I was convinced it wasn't good despite folk around me trying to reassure me. This lump terrified me............... I thought, "God help me" You see, we all like to think we are in control; it is a very human thing. To have certain things around you and a certain routine, so when you are diagnosed with something like cancer, it turns your world upside down and affects all around you, and you lose control. You are at the mercy of endless appointments with all sorts of specialists. You find yourself spending hours on the internet looking up certain words and procedures that you don't understand and then frightening yourself more.

You ask, why me? What have I done? Am I being punished, was it something in my diet, or should I have lost some of that weight? Who knows? You realise when pondering this; that it doesn't matter how you got here, you are here. And this is what you have to face. I was scared but managed to talk myself around. I will add that I do have faith and prayed like mad. And so, the journey:

I saw the GP quickly and, by 15 December, had seen a breast consultant who referred me for tests. Ultrasound, biopsy, and mammogram. By 20 December, I was informed that it was Grade 3, 3cm carcinoma with positive lymph nodes. I was devastated but to be honest, I had so much else going on in my life with a sick, elderly parent who I was solely reasonable for. I put all my issues in boxes in my mind and only dealt with the ones that needed dealing with at that time (if that makes sense).

My treatment plan was as follows: · Neo-adjuvant FEC/Docetaxel Chemotherapy (3 x FEC & 3 X Taxotere) · Lumpectomy · and radiotherapy. I was very nervous about the chemotherapy but managed to have all the prescribed doses. I did suffer from bouts of tiredness and considerable muscle/leg pain.

During the cycles of chemotherapy, when I was feeling quite well, I did work which I am sure helped with my mental health. I was told after chemotherapy that I had had a very good response, and the tumour had reduced from 3cm to 15mm.

The guidewire lumpectomy was successful, showing no residual disease, and, following the chemotherapy, none of the 13 lymph nodes had any cancer left in them. Radiotherapy, I didn't like. I think because it was every day for 3 weeks and my skin did burn.

After all this, I was very curious about how/where why Triple Negative? I did some research regarding genetics and asked if I could be tested. I was very lucky that they agreed to this. Through testing, we found out I had the faulty BRAC2 gene and was then offered more options. So, in 2012, I went on to have my ovaries and fallopian tubes removed and then a double mastectomy with DIEP reconstruction. (This was quite a massive operation, but I was back to work within 6 weeks, so I feel I did ok).

The great thing was that my daughters were able to be tested for the gene. One had it, the other not. That was very difficult, and I felt very guilty, which was ridiculous but very emotive.

And in a nutshell, that was cancer for me. However: I am now 60! I do think about it. I like to think I can help people and try to take away their worries, but we all worry from time to time. Before COVID, I volunteered at Broomfield Hospital Chelmsford to see ladies who were diagnosed with cancer and about to have surgery for reconstruction. The idea being they could look at my breasts and ask whatever questions they wanted. This was done as a group and a good thing to do. It benefited me as well as the ladies I saw. I still try to take one day at a time, deal with today and let tomorrow happen.

Lisa's Story – Diagnosed 2003

I was diagnosed with triple negative breast cancer when I was 32 years old. I remember sitting on the sofa watching TV and thinking I could feel a lump on the top of my right breast as I leaned on the arm of the sofa, but I dismissed it for a while. It bugged me until I mentioned it to my husband, who said he could also feel it easily, and we agreed I should see a doctor. My GP was great and referred me straight away, and within two weeks, I was in the breast clinic having a mammogram and biopsy.

The feeling of anxiety and nausea kicked in at that GP appointment and didn't leave me until I knew what I was dealing with. Around 10 days later, I came home from work to a letter from the hospital that was quite vague – something about results being inconclusive - and asking me to go in on the following Tuesday. Immediately I knew something was wrong because this was earlier than my scheduled follow-up appointment. Unfortunately, as it was around 7 pm on a Friday evening, I couldn't speak to the hospital until Monday morning, and during the call, they remained vague but asked if anyone would be coming with me. I guess deep down. I knew what they were going to say to me when I arrived.

Typically, my memory is awful, but that day is still crystal clear – 25 November 2003. I had chosen to go to the hospital alone, and they were clearly waiting for me as I was met on arrival at the clinic and shown into a room to wait for a doctor. He was very kind and told me he was sorry to say that I had cancer and then told me that as the biopsy had literally caught a microscopic amount of cancer cells, I was going to need another biopsy immediately. It turns out that one of the samples missed the tumour altogether and took healthy cells, but thankfully one did manage to catch it – I can't imagine how different my story would be if both samples had been missed. I remember thinking to myself that maybe it wasn't a serious kind of cancer – ridiculous, really. The diagnosis was invasive ductal cancer (Not otherwise specified), ER-negative, grade 3, stage 2, with a tumour sized 2.9cm by 2.1cm. At that time, triple-negative breast cancer as a term was not used by any of the medics I met. I spent several hours being accompanied by the breast care nurse for x-rays and the biopsy, was given lots of information on breast cancer and asked to come back the next day for a meeting with my oncologist. I was due to start a week's holiday from work, so I actually went back to work after the appointment to prepare for being out of the office, blurted the news out to my boss and said that I would update her when I knew more, then went to pick up my 18-month-old son from my mum's house. I didn't tell my mum anything at that point – I wasn't able to break that to her before my husband knew. During the day, I had played it down on the phone to him as he knew I was at the hospital; I didn't want to tell him on the phone or for him to race back in the car when he wasn't thinking clearly, and as he was working a late shift, I had to wait till around 10 pm to tell him face to face. He was devastated naturally.

The following day we were back at the hospital to meet my oncologist, who was fantastic, and I really liked him. His advice was to start chemo as soon as possible, and as we had our son already, we didn't opt for saving my eggs which would have delayed it. I was booked for a bone scan two days later and started chemo the following Wednesday. Within a week, I was in active treatment. I was lucky enough to have private care through work, so I arranged to meet a private surgeon who was recommended through the hospital, but I did all of my other treatment through the NHS.

Instantly I went from a healthy person to being told I was an incredibly sick person, but I didn't feel any different – it was very surreal. However, as soon as I had a treatment plan, I felt very positive. At no point did I really think that this cancer was going to end my life, but I am a naturally optimistic person. Telling my family was the hardest thing I've ever done as I could see their fear, and there was nothing anyone could do. I spent a lot of time telling other people it would all be fine, but I did truly believe that.

It was decided I should go for adjuvant chemo – FEC – with the intent of shrinking the tumour and enabling breast-conserving surgery, so I was given 4 rounds, then had quadrantectomy (a larger type of lumpectomy) and lymph node clearance surgery, 2 more rounds of FEC, then 20 radiotherapy sessions. I responded well to chemo, and the tumour had to be tagged with a marker after 3 rounds in case it disappeared altogether before surgery. I also felt less ill with each round, which my oncologist remarked was unusual as the effects could often be cumulative. Of course, I lost my hair, but that didn't really bother me, apart from the fact that it was a very obvious sign that I was ill. I actually found being bald liberating and have often thought I'd love to shave my head for charity! Chemo mainly made me feel exhausted, sick, constipated and like I had the worst hangover of all time. I would have given anything for an anti-nausea tablet that you didn't have to eat something before taking as I just couldn't face eating anything in the first day or two, but then I would make up for it by having all my treats in a couple of days before the next chemo when I felt well again. Overall, I lost weight on chemo, which I needed to, so I wasn't concerned.

Surgery was terrifying – I had never had an operation in my life and going down for the operation was the scariest I had ever felt during the whole experience. With surgery, too, I had no doubt it would be successful, and I remember the relief on my family's face when we got back from the follow-up appointment and told them the surgeon had confirmed he got clear margins. I was surprised at the time by their reaction of sheer relief as I truly wasn't expecting him to tell us anything else.

What was important to me was to keep things as normal as possible, so I insisted on working through all of my treatment when I was well enough. Typically, I would have chemo on a Wednesday and return to work on the following Monday. My boss was amazing throughout and bought in someone to do my job, so I could stay informed and be useful when I did go in. She even arranged for us to go out for a family meal as a treat and arranged for company chauffeurs to drive me to and from my radiotherapy appointments from the office every day at the company's expense. Looking back, I probably overdid it, though, as I also had an 18-month-old son to look after, but it was important to me at the time.

After surgery, I had my last 2 FEC chemo, which was intended to mop up any remaining cells. The very last one was a challenge due to my poor veins, and for the first time, I got fed up with being poked with needles, cried, and refused to put up with it anymore. Eventually, we agreed that I would come back in two weeks and see if we were able to find a vein, which, fortunately, we did. I found radiotherapy the easiest of all of the treatments, although I was nearly always the youngest patient in the waiting room. I completed everything around July of 2004, and we headed off to Spain for two weeks to stay with my husband's family and try to forget about hospitals for a while.

The end of treatment is tough, as almost overnight, you go from being protected by an intense treatment bubble to being expected to go back to normal life. Anxiety is never far away, as every symptom could be a sign that cancer has returned. Honestly, at first, cancer invades your thoughts constantly, and it takes months and even years for that to slowly lessen, but then you notice you aren't thinking about it as often. For a while after treatment, my tolerance of what I considered insignificant was very low, which was probably a little unfair sometimes. I had to remind myself that some things do matter and deserve to be taken seriously, especially at work, but I was caught in a mindset of "nothing really matters as much as what I have been through and might have to go through again". On the other hand, it is a sense of perspective that I now have a good balance with and am forever grateful for – not much is able to stress me out these days.

In 2003, social media was not widespread, and there were no easily accessible virtual support forums as there are today. When Facebook came along, I joined a few breast cancer groups and heard Triple Negative used for the first time; it prompted me to ask my hospital to confirm that was my diagnosis. I didn't even know anyone my age with cancer, let alone Triple Negative. These days I like to try to reassure those who are newly diagnosed that there are success stories and give them hope, as there is an overwhelming amount of negativity online.

I had had a few points of new anxiety in the last 18 years when symptoms meant I had to go back for a new biopsy or bone scan. My experience has always been that I've been taken seriously and seen quickly, and fortunately, none of them has ever ended in a new diagnosis. I think I unconsciously put my career on hold after my diagnosis – I wasn't sure I could commit to anything for a while, though in the later years, I focused again and am pleased to have progressed; I have achieved where I want to be career-wise. We also never went on to have any more children, so clearly, chemo did damage my fertility. I still have numbness in my armpit from my lymph node clearance surgery and the occasional discomfort there if I forget and overdo things, but otherwise, I am fit and well.

I am grateful in a strange way for my experience, and I am very proud to have been through it. Life is so precious, and it's easy to take things for granted when you're in the everyday routine. In 2003 we literally didn't know what my outcome would be and whether I would see my son grow up. I am beyond lucky to have survived Triple Negative breast cancer and have thrived for 18 years (and counting) after it.

Alison's Story – Diagnosed in 2011

I was lying in bed early on the morning of 11 March 2011, the day of the Japanese tsunami. I was watching the news in horror. I rolled over and thought, "ouch, that hurts". Subsequent fumbling discovered a very hard lump, which felt like a lump of old concrete with jagged edges, on the side of my left breast midway between armpit and nipple. To be honest, at that stage, I really wasn't concerned at all. I'd had multiple scares in the last 17 years as I had polycystic breasts, so I had already taken many trips to the breast unit and had lots of ultrasound scans before. I honestly did not realise the difference.

A quick pathway referral to the hospital via my GP, which I went to on my own as I had no idea this one was different, completely floored me - the consultant immediately said, "I can feel two lumps", and it was at that exact moment that I knew it was cancer. One ultrasound and biopsy on each lump later, and I drove home via the supermarket car park to give myself time to collect my thoughts and just sat in my car, sobbing.

I was back at the hospital on Friday, 1 April 2011, for my results. I was terrified because I already knew. My best friend Jan came with me and held my hand. The consultant said, "well, Alison, you do have cancer. It's Triple Negative, and it is very treatable. But you will need surgery, chemotherapy, and radiotherapy.

I knew what I wanted; I wanted this tumour out of me. Now. Today. I was lucky to have BUPA via my job, so I asked if the consultant could do the operation the next day - I was so desperate to get it out. She told me she could operate the following Friday, and we booked the appointment. My friend took me to my son's house to break the news to him and his wife, then on to my mum, who was incredibly brave and positive. Then I went home to my younger son to tell him. He fell apart.

I spoke to my boss; he broke the news to my teams at work. I knew he had lost his mum to breast cancer a few years before that. As a result, he had a breast cancer specialist friend in Essex. I asked him if he would ask his friend, the wonderful Ashraf Patel, if I could talk to him for a second opinion, and of course, Ash immediately called me. I will always be immensely grateful for that conversation, and, as a result, I decided to postpone the operation. The consultant surgeon wasn't very happy that I cancelled the surgery and tried to convince me I should still go ahead, but I was determined. This all happened on the day of diagnosis - I'm not known for hanging about when a decision needs to be made!!

The following Wednesday, I met my gorgeous oncologist for the first time, Andrew Visioli. I fell totally in love despite the circumstances! That meeting was harsh - one of the first things Andrew said was, "it's probably all-around your body already in your bone marrow". I wasn't very confident I would survive this but pushed for a chemotherapy start date at the earliest time they could do, which was 13 April.

I felt totally out of control. The absolute worst bit was the waiting. I remember emailing my boss something along the lines of "nobody's doing anything, and all the time I'm waiting, this disease is spreading around my body - I can't stand this waiting". I'll also never forget what he said to me. "Alison - you won't believe me now, but I promise you the day will come when cancer won't be the first thing you think about when you wake up in the morning or the last thing that you think about before you go to sleep". He was right; I didn't believe him then - but I do now.

I was given an unusual chemotherapy called Myocet. Andrew told me this had been specifically developed to target Triple Negative breast cancer and was only available privately. I would have 3 x 3 weekly of this and then change to different chemotherapy for another 3 x 3 weekly sessions. My lovely oncologist explained that this was because, after 3 doses, the tumour would know what was coming and would find ways of dealing with it. So, to confuse the tumour, they change the chemo. Made perfect sense to me.

My memories of the chemotherapy days are rather vague now. I felt like I was living in a haze. I had the usual side effects like nausea, constipation, mouth ulcers and no strength in my body - I couldn't even walk to the end of my very small garden and back on the bad days. Very strange feeling, difficult to describe. I was a late developer, which meant I had no reaction to the chemotherapy until day 4 or 5, and then it hit me like a ton of bricks until around day 14, when I felt ok again until my next dose.

For the fourth dose, the chemotherapy was changed to cyclophosphamide, with which I had an injection in my tummy to help with neutrophils. I could not handle this at all - I wanted to hack my head off. It hurt so much, and nothing touched the pain or the sweating. I felt so ill that I called my oncologist and told him I just couldn't do that again, so he switched my last 2 sessions back to Myocet.

During all this time, I was trying to decide if I was going to have a lumpectomy or mastectomy. I was convinced I wanted both breasts off. But both my surgeon and oncologist convinced me that a lumpectomy with total node clearance was the right thing for me.

I had a couple of ultrasound scans during the chemotherapy, which was promising, and I'd had a metal marker put into the tumour at the beginning. Two weeks after I had my last session, my very good and lovely friend Kay (who had insisted on taking me to all my chemo sessions) and I headed out on a Mediterranean cruise! I was bald, bloated and had no eyelashes or brows but did I care?

It was a lovely break, but I had my surgery to look forward to on my return.

The day of the surgery was when I discovered I had high blood pressure for the first time (hardly surprising). The surgery was easy; I had such a lovely feeling when I woke up. I didn't want to wake up properly (it must have been the morphine!), and I stayed in the hospital for just one night.

The next big thing I had to look forward to was results day, 2 weeks after surgery. I was so scared. But I got the best news ever that I had a total pathologic response, and they'd found no residual cancer in my breast or nodes. Best day of my life! After that, the radiotherapy seemed like a piece of cake!

All my breast cancer treatment had finished by mid-November 2011. Moving on to October 2013, however, I developed another cancer in my leg. This turned out to be a spindle cell soft tissue sarcoma for which I received limb-sparing surgery on 4 January 2014, followed by 7 weeks of daily radiotherapy.

I'm now approaching my 11th diagnosis anniversary for breast cancer, and I have just passed my 8th anniversary for sarcoma. I'm still "no evidence of disease". I really hope this gives newly diagnosed ladies hope for the future.

Angela's Story – Diagnosed 2010

I was diagnosed with grade 3, stage 3 Triple Negative in 2010 after finding a pea-sized lump in the shower. The tumour was 4.4cm with 4/15 positive lymph nodes and lymphovascular invasion (LVI). After genetic testing (I do not know my family history as I'm adopted), it was discovered I had a VUS (Variant of Unspecified Significance) in the Brca 1 gene, and there was not enough data to say what impact this might have or not, so I was not offered prophylactic surgery.

I had a lumpectomy, then 10 days later found out they did not get clear margins. I was offered another lumpectomy but refused and had a mastectomy the next day.

I was a 42-year-old single parent with my oldest away at university, and my other children, 10 and 13, were at home with me. I was also self-employed as a registered childminder.

I took 2 weeks off after my mastectomy. These were the worst two weeks of my life, as I googled constantly! I had to stay strong for my children, so that is what I did. However, at night when they were in bed, the tears flowed. I felt so alone and scared. My adoptive parents had both died of cancer 2 years earlier, both being diagnosed 3 weeks apart in April. My mother passed away in July and my father in December. I had no other family, and my children's father was a nut job and not around!!

I went back to work after the 2 weeks off, and I have to say this was the best thing I could have done, as it stopped me from dwelling on things. Plus, I was not entitled to any benefit due to being self-employed. I refused to let cancer take my home and business from me, but by the end of the day, I was exhausted. My 13-year-old would make me dinner while I lay on the sofa and napped. Yup, beans on toast, soup, or chicken nuggets……. I wasn't fussed, all tasted the same anyway!

I had 6 x 3 FEC-T chemo (3 weekly) at the local hospital oncology unit, a 5-minute drive from my house. I was lucky enough to have it on a Friday so that I had the weekend to recover a little. FEC was awful to me, I would vomit every hour for 48 hours after each dose, and the stomach cramps were horrible. It was a lot easier as there was no nausea. All doable, though.

My hair was so long I could sit on it, but I had it cut into a short bob; then, 13 days after my first chemo, I shaved it off. My son could not look at me, and my heart ached. He used to sit and play with my hair, and now it was gone. I had a wig, but my first chemo was in June, and the wig was horrible and hot. So, I wore buffs and bandanas instead, and once my son was ok with my bald head, I wore nothing.

After chemo, I had 20 rads over 4 weeks. The hospital was in Edinburgh, which was a 40-minute drive away, they gave me appointments in the afternoon, so I could drop my 3 little ones at nursery, run through, get zapped and go back to pick my nursery and school kids up. Radiotherapy made no change to my skin, so that was a bonus.

Treatment ended, and I decided to stay flat, as I could not leave my children alone, and I was ok with how my scar looked. However, 4 years later, I was finding it very difficult to find bras to fit. I was a 32g and had a size 9 prosthetic. All bras had an underwire and dug into my scar, and my prosthetic stuck out at the top and pulled away from my skin with the weight... not a good look.

So, with my children being a bit older and my daughter finishing university, I opted for DIEP reconstruction. Unfortunately, while checking for viable tummy blood vessels, they found a 6cm mass on my ovary, and I was taken off the DIEP list and put on the gynae list. Had a keyhole salpingo-oophorectomy and found it to be a cyst, WOOP!

Due to a friend having complications with her DIEP at that time, I changed my mind and decided an implant would be a better option for me. I spoke to my surgeon, and we agreed to go for fat transfer to soften the radiated area, then expander followed by an implant. In total, this took about a year but was more doable for me as it meant I did not need time off work.

I had 3 lots of fat transfer from my inner and outer thighs, ouch, then expander with 100mls of saline added, then I would go every few weeks to get 50mls of saline added until I had 460mls, very ouch. I had an expander out and a teardrop implant in. I then had reduction and uplift and have ended up a 32d. I refused nipple reconstruction/tattoo and opted to get my scar tattooed with flowers myself instead.

I have been finished with surgery for nearly 6 years and am happy with the way I look.

All I have had since the end of treatment is an annual mammogram on my non-cancer breast every year for the last 10 years. I saw my consultant up to year 5, then was signed off and have had the results of each mammogram in the post since.

My life has been fantastic since finishing treatment. Few ups and downs the first few years until I found my "new me", and then life settled down. In 2010 I started the first UK Triple Negative Group on Facebook, then I met a man 8 years ago, someone to share my weekends with and go out to dinner/gigs/holiday with. I'd been single for 9 years and liked my own space, but cancer made me feel lonely! I have seen my children grow up, watched them finish university, and danced at my daughter's wedding, but most of all, I've become a granny to the most amazing little girl, who makes my heart melt! I've also free fall abseiled off the Forth Rail Bridge (165ft), which my great grandfather helped build, had 22 tattoos, including my chest scar, and I've been on lots of fantastic holidays abroad, including 3 weeks touring Europe, one-year backpacking on trains, another on the back of a motorbike, and I did yoga on a beach in Cuba. I've gone around music festivals on Scottish islands, sleeping in my car and sampling all the island gins and been fly fishing with casting for recovery. I've had a body cast taken for a breast cancer awareness exhibition that toured the UK and bought myself a motorbike, which I had to give up riding due to a wee neck issue, but that was fine. Still a goal I achieved! I've paid off my mortgage and don't work too hard anymore. Still full time, but fewer hours! And lastly, I found burlesque dancing, which has given me the biggest body confidence boost ever. Before cancer, I wouldn't go topless on the beach or dance. Now I have been in 2 dance shows and have whipped my bra off in both and stood proud in front of over 200 audience members. To celebrate my 11th "cancerversary", and during the lockdown, I also rescued chickens and am now a crazy chicken lady!

2010 is a very distant memory, and life after cancer has been very good. Even in 2020, although it played havoc on life and stopped my holidays, I found so much beauty in the wee village I live in, with walks that I had never done before.

Before cancer, I was super healthy, was not overweight, went to the gym every day, did not drink/smoke/eat meat and breastfed my 3 children for over a year each.

I believe stress is caused by cancer, so I try to live as stress-free as I can and have as much fun as I can. I don't worry about the little things. If I want something, I get it. I don't have lots of income, I only work so that I can go on holidays, and I book everything myself instead of a travel agent, it's more of an adventure that way!

After cancer, did I change anything? Yes, I did. I now drink gin, wine, and cocktails!

So, my advice is everything in moderation; give up nothing! Eat the cake, chocolate, sweets, anything you fancy. At the end of the day, you have to enjoy the "new you" and not live in dread eating raw kale and watercress burgers for the rest of your life!

CHAPTER 30

WEBSITES AND USEFUL INFORMATION

For reliable research and help, please make sure you visit reputable websites (in no particular order):

Cancer Research UK - https://www.cancerresearchuk.org/

Breast Cancer Now - https://breastcancernow.org/

Macmillan Cancer Support - https://www.macmillan.org.uk/

Prevent Breast Cancer - https://preventbreastcancer.org.uk/

Team Verrico - https://www.teamverrico.org/

Predict Cancer Tool - https://breast.predict.nhs.uk/tool

UK Facebook group for Triple Negative
https://www.facebook.com/groups/TripleNegativeBreastCancerTNBCsupport/

Specific Information:

Citizens Advice Bureau – free help for financial and legal matters - https://www.citizensadvice.org.uk/

Government-backed website offering free help and guidance for benefits, money troubles, savings, pensions, work etc. - https://www.moneyhelper.org.uk/en

List of Travel Insurance companies for patients with a pre-existing medical condition (Government-backed website) - https://www.moneyhelper.org.uk/en/everyday-money/insurance/use-our-travel-insurance-directory

Campaign for free Dental Care for Cancer Patients just requires you to sign the campaign (no money required) - https://www.change.org/p/free-dental-treatment-for-cancer-patients-change-the-law

Know Your Lemons campaign (they are always looking for volunteers and also have a great app you can download) - https://knowyourlemons.org/

Cancer Support UK provides support and also chemo kits - https://cancersupportuk.org/

Website specialising in headscarves, beanies, turbans etc. https://www.annabandana.co.uk/

A US-based private company providing Genetic Testing - https://www.color.com/

Flat Friends - website and Facebook Group specifically for anybody wishing to remain flat after a mastectomy - https://www.flatfriends.org.uk

Mummy's Star – Facebook Group supporting pregnancy through cancer - https://www.facebook.com/MummysStar

Advice on hair and dollies that have hair on one side and none on the other (very cute looking and great for helping younger children understand hair loss) - https://www.facebook.com/CancerHairCare

Younger Breast Cancer Network UK – a Facebook group for ladies diagnosed with breast cancer under the age of 45 - https://www.facebook.com/YoungerBreastCancerNetwork

Support group for those diagnosed with BRCA1 and BRCA2 https://www.facebook.com/groups/1654418088135698/?ref=share

DIEP Reconstruction UK Facebook group for ladies considering a DIEP reconstruction - https://www.facebook.com/groups/562769707265849

Hair in Recovery by Racoon International – Hair extensions specifically for cancer patients or those with hair loss - https://racooninternational.com/hair-in-recovery/

Paxman Scalp Cooling Group – Facebook group (worldwide)
https://www.facebook.com/groups/285881595379700

Knitted Knockers – a group of ladies who knit prosthetics for mastectomy patients - https://www.facebook.com/knittedknockersuk

Pillow Pals – offering free heart-shaped mastectomy pillows to cancer patients

https://www.facebook.com/pillowpalsmastectomypillow

Drain Dollies – stylish bags for drains after surgery - https://www.facebook.com/draindollies

Look Good, Feel Better – an amazing charity that runs workshops at a local hospital to help you look good when undergoing cancer treatment - https://www.facebook.com/LookGoodFeelBetterUK

Maggies – providing support to cancer patients - https://www.facebook.com/maggiescentres/

Natural Image Wigs – shops around the UK and also online to purchase wigs - https://www.naturalimagewigs.co.uk

Tattoos for a Week – nipple/areola temporary tattoos - https://www.tattooforaweek.com

CHAPTER 31

GLOSSARY / ABBREVIATIONS

AC	Chemotherapy: Adriamycin (also known as Doxorubicin) and Cyclophosphamide
ADJUVANT THERAPY	Refers to treatment after surgery (for example, if you have surgery and then chemotherapy/radiotherapy – this is called Adjuvant Therapy)
ANC	Ancillary Node Clearance (where they remove all nodes from under your arm)
ANTIEMETIC	A general term for any drug that helps with nausea during treatment
BCN	Breast Care Nurse
BENIGN	Not cancerous
BISPHOSPHONATES/ ZOLEDRONIC ACID/ ZOMETA	Typically given to ladies who are post-menopausal after chemotherapy to help strengthen bones and to prevent spread to bones. Normally given every 6 months by infusion for 3 years but can be given weekly.
BRCA 1 or 2	BReast CAncer gene (a mutated gene carried by some families

	giving a greater risk of developing cancer)
CAPE	Chemotherapy in tablet form - Capecitabine
CARBO	Chemotherapy: Carboplatin
CLEAR MARGINS	During a lumpectomy, a surgeon must achieve clear margins (typically only 1mm) from the cancer cells to healthy tissue.
CPR	Complete pathological response (i.e., all cancer has gone) – the correct medical term is written as pCR (complete pathological response).
DCIS	Ductal carcinoma in situ. Pre-cancerous cells found in the lining of the breast ducts and have not "invaded" the breast tissue. The cells may or may not become cancerous.
DIEP	A type of breast reconstruction (after mastectomy) that uses your tummy fat and nerves to create breast(s)
DX	Diagnosis
DMX	Double Mastectomy
EC	Chemotherapy regime: Epirubicin and Cyclophosphamide

FEC	Chemotherapy regime: Fluorouracil, Epirubicin and Cyclophosphamide
GRADE	1-3 – Describes how quickly the cells are growing/dividing (3 being the most aggressive)
HICKMAN	A Hickman line is typically on your chest area (sometimes your arm) to administer chemotherapy instead of a cannula. Blood can be taken from it as well.
IMMUNO	Immunotherapy (a different treatment rather than chemotherapy)
INVASIVE BREAST CANCER	Cancer that has spread from the original location (milk ducts or lobules) into the surrounding breast tissue and possibly into the lymph nodes and other parts of the body. Invasive ductal cancer begins in the milk ducts. Invasive lobular cancer begins in the lobules of the breast.
Ki67	Will show on some lab reports and is the speed at which cells are multiplying/proliferating (with up to 10% being low, 20% being medium and anything

	over that being the quickest growth – Triple Negative tumours often have a Ki67 of over 70%.
LD	A type of breast reconstruction (after mastectomy) that uses your latissimus dorsi muscle in your back and brings it to the front to create a breast – typically with implants
LESION	Area of abnormal tissue
LUMPECTOMY	Also known as a Wide Local Excision or WLE. This is a breast-conserving surgery to remove the cancer tumour(s).
LYMPHOEDEMA	Swelling due to poor draining of lymph fluid that can occur after surgery to remove lymph nodes or after the radiation therapy to the area. Most often occurs in the upper limbs (arm, hands, or fingers) but can occur in other parts of the body.
LYMPHOVASCULAR INVASION (LVI)	Lymphovascular Invasion – When cancer cells spread by the blood vessels (not to be confused with lymph nodes. This is a different thing altogether.
MALIGNANT	Cancerous

MARKER	Sometimes put in at the same time as a biopsy is taken. The marker is not bigger than a grain of rice but shows on scans and can guide surgeons to the tumour (or indicates where the tumour was if the chemotherapy has killed all of the cancer).
MASTECTOMY (SMX or DMX)	The removal of the breast (or breasts) to remove the cancer and surrounding skin. It can be accompanied by immediate or delayed reconstruction, or ladies can opt to stay flat without any reconstruction. SMX – single mastectomy and DMX – a double mastectomy.
METS	Metastatic cancer, i.e., has spread to other areas of the body
MX	Mastectomy
NECROSIS	An area of skin that dies (can happen after surgery)
NED	No Evidence of Disease (i.e., the chemotherapy has removed all the cancer)
NEOADJUVANT THERAPY	This refers to any treatments, i.e., chemotherapy or radiotherapy BEFORE surgery.
NEOPLASIA	Abnormal growth

NEUTS	Neutrophils. Before chemotherapy, your blood is tested to ensure you have enough white blood cells "neuts" to go ahead with the treatment.
NEUTROPENIC	When your blood hasn't made enough cells to fight off infections so giving chemotherapy could be dangerous, and/or you're at risk of developing an infection.
NODES	Lymph nodes – normally under the arm, but there are nodes all over the body
NODE INVOLVEMENT	Cancer cells are seen in the lymph nodes after they're removed. Sometimes seen on ultrasounds, but the presence of cancer cells must be confirmed by a laboratory.
OOPHORECTOMY	Removal of ovaries (usually with tubes) to reduce risk
ONC	Oncologist
PAC / PAX	Chemotherapy: Paclitaxel
PARP INHIBITORS/ PARPS	A class of targeted therapy drugs that block an enzyme involved in DNA repair (called PARP enzyme).

pCR	A medical term - Pathological complete response (i.e., no cancer left after treatment) is also sometimes referred to by non-medical people as CPR complete pathological response.
PICC	A PICC line is a line (usually put in your arm) for chemotherapy to be administered instead of a cannula. Blood can also be taken from it.
PORT	Portacath or Power Port – A device inserted under your skin that is accessed via a needle to take blood and give you chemotherapy through.
PRIMARY TUMOUR	The original cancer or a new cancer
PROPHYLACTIC MASTECTOMY	A mastectomy is taken as a preventative measure, i.e., removing breasts where there hasn't been any cancer or removing both breasts after breast cancer.
RADS	Radiotherapy
RECURRENCE	Return of cancer. Local recurrence is the return of cancer to the same breast and can be

	linked to the previous cancer histologically.
SE	Side effects
SECONDARY TUMOUR	Secondary tumours are the same type of cancer as the original (primary) cancer. For example, cancer cells may spread from the breast (primary cancer) to form new tumours in the lung (secondary tumour). The cancer cells in the lung are just like the ones in the breast. This can also be referred to as secondary cancer.
SKIN SPARING MASTECTOMY	Where the breast is removed but keeps intact as much of the skin that surrounds the breast as possible, this skin can then be used in breast reconstruction to cover a tissue flap or an implant instead of having to use skin from other parts of the body.
SNB	Sentinel Node Biopsy – usually carried out at the start of treatment to see if your nodes are affected. Sentinel nodes are the front-line nodes.

STAGE	1-4 – Describes the size of tumour, whether nodes are involved and if there's spread
SMX	Single Mastectomy
T	Chemotherapy: Taxane, either Paclitaxel or Docetaxel
TN OR TNBC	Triple Negative or Triple Negative Breast Cancer. Breast cancer that is estrogen receptor-negative, progesterone receptor-negative and HER2/neu-negative
WLE	Wide Local Excision – also known as a Lumpectomy

ABOUT THE AUTHOR

Born within the sound of Bow Bells in London to a racing driver father and an opera singer mother, life was never going to be ordinary or dull for Michele. At the age of two weeks, she was taken to watch her father race at Silverstone and from there, travelled the world with her parents and brother.

Surprisingly, considering her mother was in the Arts, Michele was urged to have an academic career and in her mid-20s, she went to university and began a successful and long career in Human Resources. Despite that, and to let off steam, she was in a dance group in the late 1970s travelling the country and also followed in her father's footsteps by racing one of his cars.

When diagnosed with Triple Negative Breast Cancer in 2016, she re-evaluated her stressful job and since then has dedicated her time to helping cancer patients by raising funds, helping others with the same type of cancer, and starting a campaign to change the law so cancer patients have free dental care.

In late 2021, Michele was diagnosed with a completely unconnected bladder cancer which is so rare that she's only number 48 in the world with it. Despite this, Michele's outlook remains positive and thankful for a glass of red wine and laughter! Married for over 20 years to her soul mate, Can, they now live in Manchester with their daughter, Katya, who is studying to be a professional dancer.

Ingram Content Group UK Ltd.
Milton Keynes UK
UKHW020204120723
424918UK00010B/81